End your fight with

dieting, ~~scales,~~
~~bingeing, guilt,~~
~~rules~~

Food

End your fight with

~~dieting~~, ~~scales~~,
~~bingeing~~, ~~guilt~~,
~~rules~~

Food

How to change your eating habits for good

Claire Turnbull

ALLEN&UNWIN
AUCKLAND · SYDNEY · MELBOURNE · LONDON

This book's intention is to provide information and education
on how to improve your relationship with food and yourself.
It is not intended to be a substitute for professional
advice, diagnosis or treatment. The information is not
intended for the use of someone in active eating disorder
treatment. Always seek the advice of a professional.

First published in 2025

Text © Claire Turnbull 2025

Allen & Unwin
Level 2, 10 College Hill, Freemans Bay
Auckland 1011, New Zealand
+64 (9) 377 3800
auckland@allenandunwin.com
www.allenandunwin.co.nz

83 Alexander Street
Crows Nest NSW 2065, Australia
+61 (2) 8425 0100

A catalogue record for this book is available from
the National Library of New Zealand.

EU Authorised Representative: Easy Access System Europe,
Mustamäe tee 50, 10621 Tallinn, Estonia,
gpsr.requests@easproject.com

ISBN 978 1 991006 80 6

Design and illustration by Megan van Staden
Set in Söhne
Printed and bound in Australia by the Opus Group

3 5 7 9 10 8 6 4 2

MIX
Paper | Supporting
responsible forestry
FSC
www.fsc.org
FSC® C001695

To my mum and dad, who have inspired me
to show up, be brave, learn from the hard
things, try my best and, in doing so, make
a difference to the lives of others.

You will always be my heroes.

Contents

Introduction

I f you're sick of diets, over those 12-week challenges, and done with the intense feeling of disappointment when, once again, you weren't able to stick to the food, fitness or wellbeing plan you'd hoped would be 'the answer', then this book is for you.

Lying awake at night running through what you have eaten during the day and berating yourself for the doughnut/cookie/cake/chips/cheese/wine you 'promised' yourself you wouldn't have is no way to live. Nor is counting calories, obsessively tracking your macros, always weighing your food, or judging the success of your week by the number on the scales.

Quite honestly, it shouldn't be so complicated to feed your body. Yet somehow, it has become so damn hard. How is it that you can seemingly sort out other parts of your life, yet food is so challenging?

Navigating the mixed opinions, conflicting advice and false promises is perhaps the most challenging part of it all: the way it makes you feel about yourself when you just can't seem to manage your eating, or the shape and size of your body, however hard you try. Frankly, it's depressing. And then there is the guilt, the shame and the self-blame that go hand in hand with it. Made worse by the fact that you may feel like you're the only one who is dealing with this, and no one else really understands what it is like to be in a constant battle with yourself and the way you eat.

I can promise you, though, you are not alone. And, more importantly, you don't have to continue to live like this. I get it. I really do. And I am here to help you. In this book I will be sharing my story about the destructive relationship I had with both food and myself for over 20 years. I will then help you to explore *your* story and help you get to the bottom of why you eat the way you do and why you feel the way you do about yourself.

From there I will help you reprogram your relationships with food and yourself, sharing the best of everything I have learnt both professionally and from my own personal journey. My hope is that this book will help you take a large step, and maybe even a large jump, towards ending the battle between food and yourself once and for all.

'Life is too short to spend another day at war with yourself.'

— Ritu Ghatourey

I want to help you on your journey to nourish your body inside and out, so that you can look, feel and function at your best *without* a dieting mindset, restriction, or unrealistic rules around food. You should be able to enjoy a glass of wine with your friends, savour the occasional custard square, and not feel like you always have to order the 'healthiest' option on the menu. **There is room for all food as part of a balanced way of eating and living.**

My story

Growing up, I had a messy and complicated relationship with myself, and with food.

To the disbelief of people who know me now, as a young child I was quiet, massively lacked self-confidence and had no real friends. I had buck teeth, no sports skills, terrible skin covered in eczema; I struggled with dyslexia and felt like I never fitted in. It was like no one wanted to know me or be around me, so I just wanted to be invisible and disappear. So much so that I distinctly remember lying in bed some nights praying that I wouldn't wake up in the morning.

Having two brothers and only ever playing with them and the boys across the street, riding on BMXs and climbing trees, I learnt how to be around boys but didn't know how to behave around girls, and as such became an easy target to be picked on in the playground for being different. As you and I both know, children can be cruel, and words can cut deep.

My poor mum used to have to prise me off finger by finger to the teachers every day to get me to go into the school. She would then leave work at lunchtime and drive by my school to see if I was still standing in the playground all alone. Ten times out of ten, I was.

I moved primary schools multiple times in the local area where I grew up in the UK, but it never got any better. It was always a process of counting down the minutes until pick-up time when I'd get a break from the overwhelm I felt from being at school all day and hating myself for being me.

—————

When it came to the food side of things, that also wasn't plain sailing. I was a very fussy child, living on beetroot, cottage cheese and potatoes (let's be fair here, it could have been worse) and generally making my mum's life difficult when it came to eating.

My mum always appeared to be on some kind of diet. Restrictive diets were all the rage in the '80s, after all. From WeightWatchers to Slimmers World and the 'hip and thigh diet' books, it was normal to see food scales always on the bench in the kitchen. For my mum to be tracking and calculating every mouthful of food she ate was just a way of life, as was her mood being influenced by the number on the scales. She would constantly 'body check' herself, commenting on the size of her legs and stomach, putting herself down for the way she looked.

On several occasions I remember going to WeightWatchers with my mum, sitting next to her and entertaining myself while the session was going on. But I was never really just entertaining myself. I was listening, watching and absorbing what I now believe to be the utter madness going on all around me. Everyone, one by one, was weighed and then publicly congratulated — or not — based on the number on the scales. Gold stars for weight loss; even more gold stars for the 'winner of the week'; and a 'never mind' comment when the number stayed the same. A sad or disappointed look was the feedback when the number went *up*, and you needed to 'try harder' the next week.

After the scale shame came the education: 'count this', 'weigh that', 'this is good', 'this is bad', 'do this', 'don't do that' . . . on and on it went. This was just so normal in the '80s — an acceptable way to try to change the shape and size of your body.

I remember leaving a session one time when my mum had gained weight. She looked utterly heartbroken. She then beat herself up for the result, which could only have been 'her fault' and nothing to do with it being normal for your weight to go up and down. It ruined her week.

I was confused, I have to say. **How could a number change how you feel about yourself?**

Then one day, when I was about nine or ten, I remember taking the copy of the thick blue 'hip and thigh diet' book I had seen so many times out of the cupboard in our front room and reading it. As well as photos of a very slim, fit middle-aged lady in a very tight neon leotard with a sweatband on her head, there were meal plans. Calorie-counted meal plans, and rigidly strict. And with these plans right in front of me, I decided to see if I could start doing this myself.

And so my messy journey began.

I reduced the size of my breakfast, started having less lunch, turned down food when I was offered it, and to the best of my ability tried to eat less at dinner. I felt like I was winning; like I was in control. I felt like this game of counting calories was something I was good at, something I could do, and the scales fuelled my progress.

It is strange because, in hindsight, I did not set out on my journey initially to lose a lot of weight — but it didn't take long for that to change. People started to notice me. They started to comment on my weight loss, praising me and saying I looked good, which fed my desire to continue. Maybe this was the way to be seen and understood? Maybe if I looked different, dressed differently or behaved differently, people would finally accept me?

But then things got out of hand.

In the years that followed, the obsession grew and so did the weight loss. Within a couple of years my initial food rules had blown up into a full-scale eating disorder. My periods had stopped, I was hiding in baggy clothes, and people had gone from praising me to commenting on how terrible I looked. My mum often cried about how unwell I was, begging me to eat.

My poor, incredible parents who have always been there for me no matter what. What I put them through!

By the time I was 12 and at senior school I had finally made a few friends and started to feel some level of acceptance. But my unhealthy food habits were already deeply entrenched. I was absolutely using food to try to manage how I felt and to try to feel more in control of my life. I used to throw away my lunch, tell my friends' parents I had eaten at home, then tell my mum I had eaten at a friend's house. I made up all sorts of excuses and lies to avoid eating.

Then something else happened. Sleepovers with friends started in my mid-teens — and so did the 'midnight feasts' we'd have. Trips to the newsagent (dairy) after school also became more common when I had my own money and more independence around food. Following years of avoidance, came eating. Lots and lots of eating.

The next step was bingeing. It started with buying two chocolate bars instead of one, having a whole packet of crisps (chips) instead of a handful like my friends, and ordering extra-large ice creams. I just couldn't seem to stop myself. It was like a set of floodgates had opened and my brain was telling me — without any control of my own — to eat, eat and eat some more.

While there is a notion that bingeing is 'comfort eating', in my experience it is more a form of 'punishment eating' or self-abuse. After all, you don't feel good about it, or about yourself, before, during or after the whole experience. What's 'comforting' about that? Bingeing is often simply a pattern that you develop to help manage difficult thoughts and feelings. It was something I got very accustomed to.

What followed was years of a chaotic, horrible cycle of restricting and secretly bingeing: trying to eat nothing, then gorging myself and feeling like I had absolutely no ability to stop. I wasn't in control of what I was eating anymore. Far from it — food was controlling me. I hated it and, even more, I hated myself for not being able to control it. My relationship with food had become very messed up.

Then something terrible happened.

I had recently completed the Duke of Edinburgh tramp with four of my friends: Jenny, Hannah, Katherine and Alisha. We returned home exhausted and dirty but feeling heroic from our achievement. We got back to school, into the swing of things for a while, but then one evening, our home phone rang and my mum passed it to me. It was one of the other mums.

There came words that I will never forget.

'I am sorry to let you know that Alisha has died. She committed suicide.'

I dropped the phone and fell to the floor.

I was 17 years old.

She was 17 years old.

This was something you rarely saw in the papers or on TV back in the '90s. This was something that didn't seem to ever happen. So how could it have happened to someone I knew?

I then had to call Jenny; the hardest conversation I have ever had in my life. She had known Alisha since primary school.

Alisha was the most incredible girl. So smart, so talented, and so loved. She was a house leader at school, great at sports and an incredible musician; but maybe the pressure to live up to her own magic was too much for her. That's something we will never know. On the day of the funeral, I remember standing next to the hearse outside the church looking at her coffin and thinking to myself: *My god. She had no idea how much people loved her. She had no idea how many people would have listened to her and been there to help her.*

In the weeks that followed, Jenny and I spent a lot of time together, walking, talking and crying. One day when we were sitting on the floor in her room, her on the left, me on the right, I remember her saying: 'You have to start eating again — you have to sort yourself out, because if you die, too, I will never ever forgive you.'

She was so cross with me. She was so angry at what I was doing to myself, and she sure as hell wasn't going to let me forget that conversation.

So I started trying to eat 'normally' again, at least in public. I started trying to eat breakfast, have my lunch at school and not be so weird about food when I was at Jenny's house — actually eating dinner and not pretending I already had. It seemed fine for a while, but as my clothes started to get tighter my secret bingeing got worse and I just felt absolutely horrible. My daily obsession with the scales continued, my body checking got obsessive and, all in all, things felt like a disaster.

Then the *next* phase of problems began. At one of our girly 'nights in' I ate so much I felt sick, so I went to the bathroom and out the food came. It felt bad, but also good at the same time. Throwing up was horrible, but somehow the guilt of bingeing wasn't so bad afterwards. The food was gone from my body, after all.

It happened again, and again. A pattern began to emerge, and I just couldn't seem to make it stop. From throwing up after big meals and at girls' nights, I went to throwing up after every meal, snack or nibble in between. It was out of control.

I knew it wasn't right and part of me wanted it to stop, but I just couldn't. After about a year, I remember going into the bathroom, looking in the mirror and telling myself: Not today. You can eat well today. You can eat normally today. You won't binge today.

But I couldn't do it. I could never do it.

I felt like I let myself down every single day, and I began to hate myself because I obviously didn't have the willpower to control what I was doing, when, surely, I should! I had controlled my eating before, so why couldn't I do it now?

———

After finishing school at 18 I planned to go to university. What was I going to do? Coming from a medical family — my dad a doctor, my mum a nurse, and one of my brothers having studied pharmacy, then medicine — a future for me in health felt like the path to follow. Medicine, physio, speech therapy and dietetics were on my shortlist. I landed a four-year full-time degree in nutrition and dietetics in Leeds in the north of England. I figured that if I could learn everything there was to know about food, maybe I could figure this thing out, sort myself out and help other people, too. So off I went to uni, with a fresh start ahead of me and a whole lot of hope that things would be different.

But, alas, my problems followed me. Now that I was in control of my own food shopping, with the addition of lots of alcohol, things got even more crazy. The restriction, bingeing and throwing-up cycle continued. I then trained to be a fitness instructor and added over-exercising and laxatives into the mix. A disaster, to say the least!

Some afternoons I would eat three family-sized bags of Maltesers at once. On others I would drink a full cup of Malibu out of a mug. Ice cream became a food I had no control over. I had a complete inability to stop eating. The day I managed to eat an entire family-sized jar of Nutella in one go, sitting on my bedroom floor, under my desk, and crying each time the spoon went in my mouth is one I will never forget. I have never felt so sick from eating and never felt more disappointed in myself for what I was doing.

In my second year of university my mental health took a turn for the worse. I was ready to give up my fight with food and with myself and just wanted it all to be over. Luckily, a friend walked into my room as I was plotting my exit and marched me down to the doctor's, which was just about to close. She stood in reception and said that she wasn't going to leave until they did something to help me.

I will never, ever forget that day.

I sat on the doctor's folded-up bed/couch with the curtain around me and said out loud for the first time in my life words that I had felt inside for a long time.

'I don't feel safe in my own company.'

I started on antidepressants, and off I went back to my life.

The suicidal thoughts did subside, but I never felt right; I still doubted my self-worth constantly. My eating issues were still there; I was still drinking too much, too often; and I still had an unhealthily obsessive relationship with exercise.

But I charged on, studied through, passed my degree with flying colours, and went off into the working world.

———

My first job was as a clinical dietitian at Arrowe Park Hospital on the Wirral peninsular where I grew up. I was working in intensive care, on the gastro wards, and running diabetes clinics. I loved it — but still didn't anywhere near love or even *like* myself.

By this point, my eating problems were so deeply entrenched into my being that I just thought this was how life would always be. Maybe I would just always struggle in this way and have to live with feelings of deep sadness and utter disappointment with myself for not being able to get myself together, in a space which was made worse because I was now a qualified dietitian and surely I should know how to manage this. Right?

Turns out, not so.

After a difficult year or so, I decided that I needed to change my scenery and try to get away from my problems — which is when I made the move from the UK to New Zealand. Because, surely, moving to the other side of the world on your own will deal with all your demons, right?!

Umm. That didn't go so well.

'Wherever you go, there you are.'
— Zen proverb

When I got here, I assured myself that this would be the time when I could start over. Surely over here I would be able to eat normally, stop bingeing, drink like a 'normal' person and be able to stop myself after one scoop of ice cream. But that didn't happen. Instead, I absolutely fell apart.

What was wrong with me, for goodness' sake? I knew my family loved me and would always be there for me. I had friends now, I had a job I was good at, so why could I not pull myself together?! I knew what I should be doing. I knew what I needed to eat. I knew what it took to be healthy and balanced.

Why couldn't I make it happen?

Finally, in 2006, when I was 24 years old, my aunty (who I was staying with at the time) suggested that I reach out for help. So, reluctantly, I booked an appointment to see a psychologist. I wish I could say it was the best thing that ever happened. But it wasn't; he wasn't the right fit for me. I still felt lost and hopeless. Luckily, though, as a health professional myself I knew that sometimes you don't always hit the jackpot first time around. I just needed to see if I could find someone who was a better fit. And after a while, I did. I found someone who helped me start my journey of recovery. Someone who helped me begin to understand myself and understand why I was eating the way I was. She showed me how I could build a better life for myself — something that at that stage I never believed was possible.

At last I was able to see that my eating issues were nothing to do with food. Instead, they were simply the way I was trying to manage difficult emotions and how I felt about myself. After all this time, I finally felt free. I could see that I was not the problem. That food was not the problem. Growing up, I had simply learnt some really unhelpful and destructive habits and behaviours that I needed to rewire to get myself into a better space.

This was not something that was taught as part of nutrition when I was studying. Back then, it was all about 'knowledge equals change' — if you know what to do, you can do it. Right? Wow. How misguided that teaching was. Those overly simplistic views are what fuelled diet mentality, guilt and shame, for me as well as for others.

From that point it took me over ten years to completely stop bingeing and throwing up. From multiple times a day, to a few times a week, to every few months, and then longer gaps. The last time I binged, I was age 34. I am now 42. Bit by bit, I got better, and learnt more about myself every step of the way. How I did that is what I want to share with you in this book.

Since the first time I reached out for help, I have been on an amazing, wild journey of self-discovery and have fully immersed myself in the study and exploration of what it is that makes us who we are, and why we eat and behave the way we do. I am extremely passionate about sharing with you, through this book, everything I have learnt over the past few decades in the hope that it can help you finally find peace with food; and simultaneously find compassion for yourself and what you have been through in your life.

———

There are so many reasons why we can struggle with ourselves and food. For me, it started with very low self-worth and a diet book that turned into an obsession. For you, it could be something completely different. If you were brought up in an abusive home, it could be that eating became a means of escapism; or that living in a larger body is what subconsciously helps you feel safe if you were violated as a child. Perhaps you were told that you were too fat and put on diets at a very young age. Or maybe you simply had to compete with your siblings or with other kids at boarding school to ensure you got your fair share of food.

Whatever your story, common themes often hold true. Restriction, overeating, body dissatisfaction, self-judgement, guilt and shame. An ugly mix that can take over your life.

My approach in this book will support you to be in the driving seat of your choices around food, no longer feeling like you need to follow a restrictive diet. I will help you to reprogram any unhelpful eating habits that are sabotaging your wellbeing goals — be it bingeing, eating when you are bored, drinking when you are stressed, picking at food when you are lonely or tired, polishing off the rest of that packet of biscuits after telling yourself you wouldn't have any because, sod it, you have 'blown it' now anyway . . . And so the list goes on.

I will be helping you to develop confidence, which will make it easier for you to make choices that help you feel good, and to reduce your reliance on willpower, especially when you are busy! I will also be helping you to work out what approach to food is right for *you*, because there really is no 'one size fits all'. Different things work for different people. **Much of this process is about learning to reconnect with yourself and allow yourself to work out what is best for you.**

As part of our journey together in this book, I am also going to be supporting you to improve your overall wellbeing, because sleeping well, moving your body, managing stress, having healthy relationships and knowing your purpose all play their part in building a healthier relationship with both food and you. Plus, all these things also help you feel and function better, which is an all-round win!

If you have picked up this book because you really just want to shift 5 kilos or drop a dress size (or three) — then yes, by addressing your unhelpful eating patterns and looking after yourself better, these outcomes may well be part of this journey. However, rather than either of those being the barometer of your success, instead, please, let it be how different you feel, how much energy you have and how much more free your mind feels when dieting no longer takes up so much head space. In both my professional and my personal experience, focusing on weight or size as your primary goal is unhelpful and messes with your mind. So, if you haven't already, **get rid of your scales**. You are not going to need them here.

I don't have all the answers and I don't know it all; but when I recovered from one of my very dark spots, I promised myself I'd spend the rest of my life helping people who struggle with their relationship with food and with themselves to find peace and a sense of joy, knowing that they can feel good again. So that's what I'm here to do. To share what I know, to share what has worked for me, so you can take the parts that work for you and during the process learn something about yourself.

Let's say goodbye to diets and focusing on weight, and move forward with a more soulful journey.

'If you change the way you look at things, the things you look at change.'

— motivational speaker
Wayne Dyer

Getting started

What lies ahead in this book is all sorts of different ideas for you to try. But, as it can be really easy to become overwhelmed by a lot of information, **please don't feel like you have to do everything in one go.** Use the suggestions in this book in a way that works for *you*. You might want to read the book from cover to cover, then come back and do some of the exercises that resonate with you. Or you might want to take things step by step as you go through. It is up to you.

The first part of the book is all about understanding your influences and how they impact your behaviour and your perception of yourself. The second part of the book looks at reprogramming your eating habits using my four-step process, which I have found works wonders! The third part covers off my Wheel of Wellbeing, looking at sleep, nourishment, movement, stress management, relationships, and meaning and purpose.

Some of you might be approaching this journey sleep-deprived, exhausted and totally overwhelmed. If this is you, feel free to read the sleep section first and get that sorted, then come back to the start and work on reprogramming your eating when you have more energy to do so.

Equally, if you are really stressed at the moment and just the thought of working on your eating habits feels too much right now, then read the stress section first and come back to the eating habit reprogramming later.

Also, I highly recommend that you **start small**. As I said earlier, you don't have to do everything all at once! Work on one thing at a time, and when you have really got to grips with that one you can move on to something else.

This book opens up the start of a new journey, and it is going to be a **process**. It didn't take you six weeks to get to where you currently are with the challenges to your health and wellbeing — so it is not going to be a six-week quick-fix to get out of there either! Give yourself time, and take the approach of this being **a journey of joy that will bring you back home to the best version of you**. The planners on my website will be a real help, and do follow me on my social channels for extra support.

'Start where you are. Use what you have. Do what you can.'

— athlete Arthur Ashe

Another hot tip you will see featured many times in this book is the value of good old **pen and paper** for writing things down — so be sure to have these at the ready as you go through the book. Writing down your goals can significantly increase the likelihood of you achieving them — by an estimated 42% in fact! And getting those swirling, often negative thoughts out of your head and down on paper helps you distance yourself from them and see them for what they are, which can be its own form of therapy. Sometimes the simplest things can be the most effective.

What is your WHY?

Here is something to ponder on as you read through this book: **Why** is it important to you that you work on yourself and take care of yourself?

Initially you might think 'to feel better', or 'to look healthier', or 'to have more energy', and the like — but I want you to dig a bit deeper and find out WHY those things matter. For example, why do you want to feel better? So you have more energy to play with your kids? To make your work life easier? To have more mental capacity to engage in friendships? To have the confidence to date again? To be fit enough to hike with your friends or do a long bike ride next year?

There is no right or wrong here, but as you venture on the journey ahead of you, it is really helpful to have a connection to something other than your body looking different. What will looking after yourself give you on a *deeper* level?

Make space

You will also need to **create space in your life** for this journey of change. I know this isn't the quick-fix/easy answer we all want to hear, but anything worth doing is worth doing well or the results won't last. Creating space can look different for us all; it might be committing to less, asking for more help, or giving up the idea that you can do it all. None of us can do everything.

To go through the process of writing this book, I had to create space. I had to say no to many social events and to some really good work and travel opportunities. I had to give up many weekends with my family and friends. I had to ask for help. But going through that process was one of the best things I have ever done. Now I am out the other side, I am able to be a better version of me both for myself and for everyone else. **The same can be true for you and the process of self-discovery and healing that is ahead of you.**

You are worth it. You deserve to take the time to do something for yourself, and also be kind to yourself on this journey. When you are the best version of yourself, who knows what is possible for you? Right?

Let's get to it.

'Take care of yourself. You can't pour from an empty cup.'

— Unknown source

Part 1

Understanding your influences

Chapter 1

The tip of the iceberg – and what's beneath the surface

When we are struggling with things in our lives, it is often *behaviour* we point the finger at. For example, with my eating challenges it appeared that the restricting and bingeing combined with drinking too much were the problems that needed to be solved.

For years upon years, I worked to solve these problems. The assumption I made was that if I just 'tried harder', used my willpower and focused a bit more, then I would be able to change my behaviour and make the problems go away. That was what all the diet books and magazines had been telling me, after all. But as you know from my story, that didn't happen. Even as a fully qualified dietitian and fitness trainer I couldn't make those changes happen.

While it might seem logical that if you 'know what to do' and just 'try harder' you'll be able to change the way you behave, and control the choices you make, that isn't how it works in real life. Knowledge and willpower are important, for sure, but on their own they are rarely enough to tackle unhelpful behaviours. This is why you end up feeling like you have failed at following the diet plan you were given or the rules you were trying to stick to — because they were overly simplistic and one-dimensional in their approach.

But *you* didn't fail. The *approach* did. You don't need to keep being more restrictive or try harder to change your behaviour; you just need to take a new, more holistic approach based on how the process of behaviour change actually works.

———————

When it comes to understanding behaviour and how to change it, I find the analogy of an iceberg useful.

What you see above the water is the tip of the iceberg, which is like the behaviour we see on the outside. With our wellbeing, these behaviours can include how we eat, how often we exercise, how we talk to ourselves, how much sleep we get, how we react to stressful situations and so on.

I like to think of behaviours as either being *helpful* or *unhelpful*.

- **Helpful behaviours** are those that support us to live our best lives, when we feel and function at our best.
  Using food as an example, helpful behaviours are balanced and realistic rather than obsessive or restrictive. This

includes things like enjoying plenty of fibre-rich vegetables in your meals because they help your body work well and can help reduce your risk of anxiety and depression. Another example is being able to stop eating when you feel you have had enough, *most of the time*.

- **Unhelpful behaviours** are those that *don't* make us feel good and, at times, might be sabotaging our overall health and wellbeing.

  Again with reference to food, some examples of unhelpful behaviours could be buying doughnuts at the supermarket every week and eating them before leaving the car park even though you don't really want them; or having a tiny, low-carb lunch and then emptying half the fridge in the evening because you are so hungry; or drinking wine every night at home on your own to manage your feelings of overwhelm and loneliness even though you have wanted to stop drinking for months because it is impacting your sleep and also costing too much. Another example is finding it hard to say no to food offered by others when you aren't hungry, because you don't want to appear rude or let someone down.

To be very clear, when it comes to behaviours, there is a reason why I have chosen the words **helpful** or **unhelpful** rather than 'good' and 'bad', especially when it comes to the topic of food. That's because the words good and bad come with loaded meaning. 'Bad' eating makes you feel like you have done something wrong by eating — which you haven't.

Also, a 'helpful behaviour' in relation to eating *doesn't* always mean you have to have salad at every meal, or always go for the alcohol-free drink options (unless you want to). **Mindfully** enjoying a slice of carrot cake from time to time or **intentionally** enjoying a glass of wine with a friend at the weekend, for example, can still be helpful behaviours when — as part of the overall balance of your life — these things fit in and make you feel good. Note the words I've highlighted here: acting *mindfully* and *intentionally* is very different to acting out of habit or obligation.

Going back to the iceberg, the — much bigger — part beneath the water is what is *influencing* our behaviours. With regard to food there are some more obvious things near the surface of the water, like our knowledge of nutrition, our cooking ability, our access to food, our budget, how active we are and how much we sleep. (I am not the only one who can't stop eating after a bad night's sleep, right?!)

Beyond the obvious, though, there are also deeper roots, which are often 'invisible' — they influence our behaviour often without us consciously realising. This includes things like our beliefs, values, habits, thoughts and emotions (which I will be going into in more detail soon).

What I learnt on my own journey is that my unhelpful behaviours are just a signpost and symptom of much deeper challenges. To change our unhelpful behaviours, we need to address the things *underneath* the tip of the iceberg. This principle applies to all unhelpful behaviours — everything from mindless phone scrolling and online shopping addiction to smoking, vaping and being passive-aggressive. You need to scratch below the surface to see what is driving these behaviours.

As for many other people, the root cause of my eating issues wasn't food; it was more about the fact that I didn't believe I was good enough and the only way I felt like I could control my life was by controlling what I ate. Beyond that, food and alcohol became my coping mechanism for difficult feelings.

My goal in this book is to help you understand more about *your* iceberg and what is driving your behaviours so you can take control

BEHAVIOUR

Habits

Values

Beliefs

Thoughts

Emotions

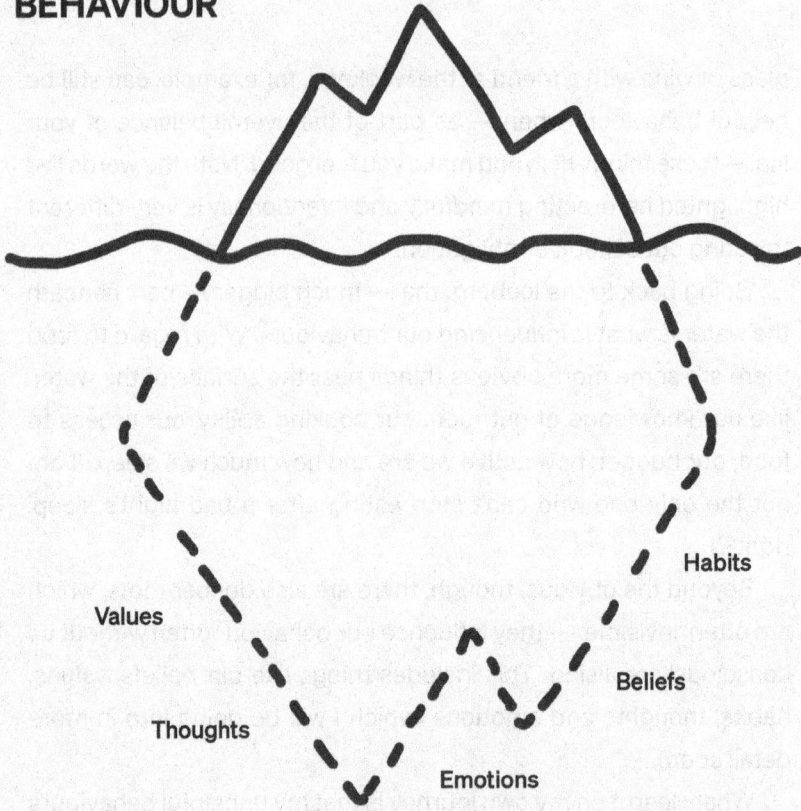

of them. I hope to help you reprogram the unhelpful ones and build helpful new ones so you can be the best version of you.

Later in this book, I will be sharing my best tips and tricks for how to make it easier to make nourishing food choices, and addressing the many other more 'obvious' influences when it comes to food, as there is still merit in that. But before we get to that part, I want to dive into the 'invisible' influences because I believe these are often missed and where magic can happen.

These 'invisible' influences are what you need to look at to be able to make lasting changes to the way you eat, as well as changing any other behaviours you want to in your life.

Beliefs

In a nutshell, your beliefs are assumptions that you have about yourself, the world and other people. They are often based on what you saw, heard, read and experienced growing up, which is why I will soon be asking you all sorts of different questions about your upbringing to start unlocking some insight for you.

As a child, you don't consciously choose your beliefs; they develop as a way for your brain to try to make sense of the information it receives from the world around you as you grow up, and, in a way, to create a form of self-protection. These beliefs are designed to help you predict what is safe and what you need to stay away from. In reality though, as you will soon see, it doesn't always work out this way!

Your beliefs essentially become part of the rule book by which you subconsciously make decisions in your life. Your beliefs influence all sorts of things in both the tip and the bottom part of your iceberg, including how you think, feel and behave. They can come across stronger and weaker at different times in your life depending on what's going on for you at the time, but they are always sitting there in the background.

Your **core beliefs** are the big ones — the ones that you believe to be completely true about yourself. Statements of these core beliefs often start with the word 'I'. These can then get **supporting beliefs** tacked on to them. Here are some examples:

- Maria: **I am no good at sport.** *There is no point trying, as I will only do badly and look stupid.*
- Elisha: **I am too fat to be successful in the workplace.** *I shouldn't apply for jobs that are too challenging.*
- Ivana: **I am smart.** *I can do well at work.*
- Sharam: **I am not good enough to find love.** *No one will accept me the way I am.*

- Fei: **I can do hard things.** *It is okay to try new things even if I fail.*
- Kerry: **I can't control myself.** *I can't consistently eat well. I can't stop drinking. I can't keep up an exercise programme. There is no point trying anymore.*
- Mish: **I can be healthy and happy.** *It's worth planning meals that make me feel good.*

You will notice that, like behaviours, sometimes these beliefs are helpful, like Fei believing she is able to do hard things in her life. Her deep sense that failure is not to be feared means that she is likely to try lots of new experiences as she goes through life.

Sometimes, however, beliefs can be incredibly unhelpful and destructive. These are often referred to as **limiting or false beliefs**. They can trigger a chain reaction of negative self-talk, eroding your worth and self-esteem and negatively impacting the direction of your life. One way this can end up being expressed is by driving you to make choices around food and alcohol that don't make you feel good and sabotage your wellbeing.

These limiting or false beliefs can be formed after big events, but equally might be formed as a result of a few words in the playground. Wherever they come from, it is important that we question whether or not they are helpful to hold on to as we progress through our adult life. Maybe these beliefs are part of what is holding us back from the life we dream of living.

Later in the book I will be helping you to rework the limiting beliefs that are holding you back. For now, I just want you to be aware that your beliefs are part of what is influencing why you eat, behave and treat yourself the way that you do.

Values

Values are, in essence, the things that really matter to us and, without us knowing, they can hugely influence our behaviour and the decisions we make. Examples of values include commitment, courage, equality, fun, health, independence, loyalty, power, security, travel, wealth, wisdom . . . and so the list goes on. Like your beliefs, your values can be heavily influenced by your environment, upbringing, culture, experience, trauma history and social circles.

I have worked with many people to help them identify their values, and it is always the most enlightening experience.

For one of my friends, her top value is *fun*, closely followed by *adventure, freedom* and *flexibility*. Knowing this made it much easier for her to see why she struggled to get into a good routine with her eating and would always be up for a drink (or six) whatever the occasion. Fun and adventure subconsciously ruled her choices. On the one hand she loved this because it made her feel like herself; but on the other she got really annoyed about it because, deep down, she wanted to get into a healthier routine and she could clearly see alcohol affecting her work, mood and sleep. It was also interfering with her close relationships and causing financial pressure.

Becoming aware of her values helped my friend to see what was impacting her behaviour. From there she was able to make some adjustments and weave in a degree of planning that still enabled *flexibility*. She also started getting more into cooking and joined a kickboxing studio, both of which she found *fun* and like an *adventure* because she was meeting new people and trying new things — while supporting her wellbeing goals at the same time.

Later (on page 263) I will be taking you through an exercise to help you figure out what your values are, but for now just be aware that values are another invisible layer driving how you behave, and are likely in some way to be influencing your behaviour.

Habits

Your brain is a prediction machine. As you go through your day-to-day life, one of its jobs is to figure out what information is worth keeping track of and what's not. When things happen repeatedly, over and over, your brain starts to see these as patterns that must be worth remembering. So, in an effort to make it as easy as possible for these things to happen, it embeds them into your subconscious as 'habits' so that they happen without you having to think about them.

As early humans evolved, habits served as a survival function by allowing us to efficiently and easily carry out routine actions. That meant we were able to free up cognitive resources (brain power) for more complex tasks or unexpected situations — which was much needed back then when you had to regularly fight for your life or be able to run away from danger very quickly to survive.

Habits provide predictability and control in our environment, which can help reduce stress from uncertainty — which, obviously, can be helpful. When it comes to things like brushing your teeth or getting up at 6 a.m. every day to walk the dog, it's good that those things happen without too much effort. Sadly though, habits can also be unhelpful: always finishing your plate despite being full, or opening the fridge the minute you walk into the kitchen even if you only came in to grab the laundry and didn't want anything to eat.

Research from Duke University in the US suggests that approximately 40% of our behaviours are habitual. That is a whopping 'invisible' influence in the submerged part of your iceberg! So if you can make your habits work in your favour rather than against you, it is possible to create profound changes in your life. Much of this book is about figuring out what your unhelpful eating habits are and how to reprogram them, so rest assured: solutions are coming.

TRIGGER

HABIT LOOP

REWARD

BEHAVIOUR

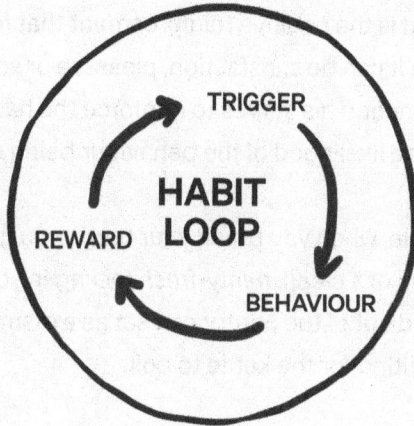

How habits form

Habits follow what is called a habit loop. It has three main parts: a trigger, a behaviour, and a reward.

- **The trigger**, also known as a cue or prompt, is what starts the habit loop off and kicks the automatic behaviour or response into action. Habit triggers can be environmental cues such as specific locations, times of day, objects, people or emotional states.

  An example of a trigger for the helpful habit of brushing your teeth is finishing your breakfast and putting your bowl in the sink or dishwasher.

  For the unhelpful habit of picking at food in the pantry, a trigger might be putting the kettle on and waiting for it to boil.

- **The behaviour**, also known as the action or response, is what you do, say or possibly even just think following the trigger. So, for the examples above, it would be brushing your teeth or eating food out of the pantry.

- **The reward** is the positive reinforcement that follows the behaviour; it can be satisfaction, pleasure or some other form of benefit. This serves to reinforce the habit loop and increase the likelihood of the behaviour being repeated in the future.

  For example, when you brush your teeth, you get the satisfaction of a *clean, minty-fresh feeling* in your mouth. Eating food out of the pantry can act as a *distraction* while you are waiting for the kettle to boil.

Where cravings come from

When it comes to food, cravings are those uncontrollable desires you experience when you feel like a prowling tiger ready to hunt down some salty chips, chocolate or anything that is packed with sugar to give you a quick energy hit. The same is common with alcohol, too. You almost feel drawn to the alcohol cupboard or fridge like you don't have a choice about it.

But where do these cravings come from?

When you think about something you want to eat or drink, or see something tasty sitting on the bench, that's a trigger for your brain to release a burst of the neuromodulator dopamine. This is a chemical that changes the electrical activity of nerve cells throughout your nervous system. While dopamine is often thought of as a feel-good hormone that acts as a buzz, there's more to it than that. One of its key functions is to activate motivation: to encourage and drive behaviour.

It works that way because the dopamine hit you get when you think about what you want to eat, drink or do soon drops back down, and then goes below your normal baseline levels. This is what creates the feeling of a 'craving'. Your body wants more feel-good

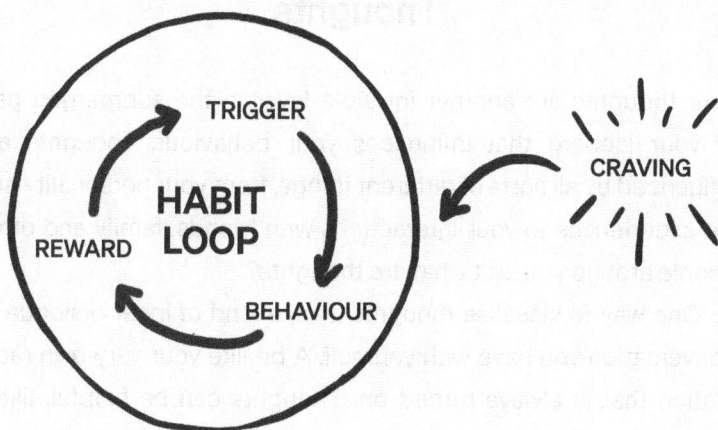

dopamine, but the low levels you now have are creating a sense of agitation in your body, a sort of pain that drives you to take action and — in the case of habits — complete the habit loop by giving yourself a reward.

When you get the reward and the habit loop is completed, the agitation stops and for a while you feel calm again. Until it kicks off *again*.

Have you ever felt that sense of agitation in your body? The feeling that drives you to the pantry, the fridge or into the petrol station to get an ice cream on your way home? It is powerful, and can feel like you haven't got conscious control over it. Which, in a way, you don't.

The added challenge here with cravings and food is that you can't practise abstinence, as is recommended with other things like gambling or drugs. Instead, you have to work to find the balance between feeding your body for nourishment and enjoyment without eating mindlessly, out of habit. More on how to do this coming up.

Thoughts

Your thoughts are another invisible layer in the submerged part of your iceberg that influences your behaviour. Thoughts are influenced by all sorts of different things, from your personality and life experiences to your interactions with friends, family and other people around you. But what *are* thoughts?

One way to visualise thoughts is as a kind of inner dialogue or conversation you have with yourself. A bit like your very own radio station that is always turned on. Thoughts can be helpful, like 'I really feel good after exercise'; or neutral, like 'I need to feed the cat'; or negative, like 'I am just going to look stupid if I go'. You might be consciously aware of some of your thoughts, or not be in tune with them at all.

While it is pretty much impossible to know how many thoughts we each have in a day, scientists suggest that it is many thousands, which is a *lot* of thoughts. Particularly when thoughts can have such a big (invisible) influence on our behaviour.

An important thing to be aware of when it comes to thoughts is that they can get stuck on repeat. When you have the same thoughts over and over, they can become beliefs. For example, say that every time you see food, see someone eating food, think about food, shop for food or go anywhere food is, you have the thought: *I have no self-control over food.* Soon enough, you will come to believe this thought to be true, even though in reality it is unlikely to be true 100% of the time. What happens then? Every time you eat more than you wanted to, you hold on to this as evidence that your belief is true and you have no control — which feeds the thought, which feeds the cycle. A cycle which I will soon be helping you break!

The most important thing of all, which I tell my children almost every day, is that **just because you have a thought that DOES NOT MAKE IT TRUE!** Thoughts are just thoughts — a bit like opinions.

They are not necessarily reality. As humans we like to have everything make sense and have meaning, so we must be mindful of the thoughts we allow to replay in our mind or they could take us away from the life we deserve. I will be helping you with this in Chapter 11 (see pages 266–273).

Emotions

Emotions arise quickly, and can occur automatically without conscious thought. As such, they — like beliefs, values and thoughts — act invisibly, in the hidden part of the iceberg, and can have a huge impact on your behaviour.

There is much debate about how to define an emotion, and about how emotions arise in the body. To keep things really simple here, it's helpful to think about emotions as being like the data your brain uses to figure out how to respond.

From an evolutionary perspective, emotions are likely to have motivated us to act in different ways to help our survival. Fear, for example, can motivate you to run away from danger, which historically would have been vital if you saw a lion or a tiger approaching. Anger, on the other hand, could motivate you to attack or defend yourself, which, again historically, would have been essential if you were being threatened by an incoming tribe wanting to take the land you relied on for your survival.

When you think about eating and drinking, what emotional states come to mind? The common ones are *sadness*, linked to eating comforting foods; and *happiness* or *excitement*, associated with celebration (often meaning alcohol, tasty snacks or indulgence of some kind). There are, however, so many more emotional states which we experience as human beings that can drive our eating and drinking in a variety of ways. *Shame, anger, fear, disgust, boredom, loneliness* and *guilt* are just a small handful of examples of emotions that drive unhelpful eating. *Relaxed, calm, balanced, content, respected* and *hopeful* are some examples of emotional states that might be more likely to drive helpful eating behaviours.

In creating a healthier relationship with food and with yourself, it is helpful to tune in to your emotional state at different times and look at how you are reacting or managing different emotions. If, for example, you notice what feels to you like loneliness, this might be a trigger for you to seek comfort in food or drink to help numb that emotion. Equally, if you feel joy and excitement, this may lead you to feel like you need to crack open a bottle of wine because, well, that's what has become a normal action for you when you feel this way.

If you have emotional triggers that play their part in unhelpful eating behaviours, you can't just avoid or ignore them — they can be huge drivers of a behaviour you are trying to change. Instead, you need to find a way to work through these challenging emotions. The aim is to get to a point when you feel you are in control of them, rather than them being in control of you. This is something we will be working through in Chapter 5.

Reflecting on what drives a behaviour

Now you know a bit more about some of the invisible influences sitting in the hidden part of the iceberg of behaviour, let's go back to a couple of our earlier examples and see what kinds of things could be driving the behaviour from below the surface.

The post-shopping doughnuts:

- Could it be that you aren't eating enough during the day and are always so hungry by the time you finish shopping that you really want something sweet to perk you up? **(habit)**

- Or is it because as a child you always had to share everything, and now you want something all to yourself without anyone else getting a look-in? Maybe you hold a **belief** that there is not enough food to go round?
- Or is it that deep down this is about you needing five minutes to yourself for the first time all week without anyone bothering you? You might have strong **emotions** of overwhelm and have a **habit** of rewarding yourself with food.

The 6 p.m. wine routine:

- Is this helping you to manage feeling stressed or lonely? **(emotions)**
- Is it the only way you feel like you connect with your partner? **(value)**
- Is it because you feel like you deserve a treat after a big day? **(habit)**

There are so many examples I could give here, but the key thing for you to see is that any frustrations you have with the way you're eating and drinking can't be glossed over with a 'one size fits all' approach that doesn't get to the root of the problem.

———

Our mission together in this book is to look at the behaviours that aren't working for you in your life, and figure out what is driving those behaviours by looking at what lies underneath them. This will give you the information you need to be able to reprogram them. We will dig deep into habits and emotions soon, and later in the book we'll do the same for values, thoughts and beliefs.

But before we go any further, *right here, right now* I would love you to do something for me — or at least make it one of your goals as you work through this book. **STOP beating yourself up.** Stop beating yourself up for not going to the gym when you told yourself you would; stop hating yourself for not following through on your diet plans or for having a third glass of wine. You have simply been doing what many of us do when we are struggling: finding a way to manage.

The judgement and shame you have no doubt been inflicting on yourself for years about the way you eat and drink will have only been driving those unhelpful behaviours and making you feel terrible about yourself. This is no way to live.

So, **give yourself a break** for being human.

Let's focus on trying to understand a bit more about what is in the underneath part of your iceberg so that you can finally find a way to manage your eating and drinking in a way that works for you.

It is time to hit the next stage of your self-discovery adventure with a positive attitude and an open mind.

KEY MESSAGE

You aren't broken — you never were. You are human.

Chapter 2

How the outside world shapes your inside world

Our journey together over the next few chapters is all about looking at the big bit of your iceberg underneath the water's surface, to see what you can find out about the different experiences you have had that might be influencing your behaviour. The focus here is on your relationship with food and how you think and feel about yourself.

The questions I ask may bring up all sorts of memories, thoughts and feelings, so **go gently with yourself** and seek support from a friend or a qualified health professional if you need to. Digging into the details of who you are and why you behave the way you do can bring up all sorts of things, but I really do believe that this step is often what gets missed — and it is where magic can happen.

I liken this approach to working on a house renovation project. If you want a quick fix, you can slap a coat of paint on the outside, put up some new curtains . . . and voilà, your house will look better for a while. But if the foundations of the house are unstable and there are cracks in the walls, the results of this quick-fix job will soon fade — especially when a storm hits. It's much the same when following a diet plan for a couple of months. You look and feel great, temporarily, and start getting compliments from your friends — but then life happens. Work gets busy, your dog/child/mum/dad/gran/ friend gets sick, the washing machine breaks, someone crashes into your car and, alas, your quick repair job doesn't stand the test of time. Your old eating and drinking patterns come back in a flash.

The reality is, though, that **there are always going to be these ups, downs, storms and challenges in your life**. They are unavoidable; part of being a human being living in this crazy modern world.

So if you are looking to properly renovate a house, you first need to look at what is going on *underneath* the house and make sure everything is stable. Without a solid base, other changes you might make are often temporary or can easily be broken. To be able to make changes to the way you eat, your relationship with food and how you think about yourself — changes that last the test of time and are able to adapt to the realities of real life — you must understand your own foundations. The things that make you who you are. The things that make you behave, eat, drink and do the things you do.

So, it is now time to get digging deep . . .

KEY MESSAGE

When you understand yourself, how you think, feel and act, it can have a profound effect on your life.

Your early years

From the moment you were conceived, your development was influenced by things outside of your control. The amount of stress your mum had to manage, how much sleep she had, as well as what she ate and drank while you were inside are just a handful of the things that will have had an impact on how your brain and body developed.

Once you were born, the environment you grew up in and the experiences you had as a young child continued to influence the way you developed. Current research indicates that the first 1000 days will have had the most impact. It is during these two and a half years that your nervous system (brain, spinal cord and nerves) is set up in a way that will best support your long-term survival in the world — based on your early environment and experiences.

If you experienced a lot of stress or trauma in those early years, this may have strengthened sections and circuits in your nervous system in particular ways — for example, by causing you to respond to threat or overwhelm by distancing yourself from (or completely suppressing) challenging emotions. This may now be reflected in your current behaviour — for example, excessive reactivity, withdrawal, defensiveness or other such coping mechanisms that you have developed to manage anything that feels threatening. Food and alcohol, as well as drugs and other substances and behaviours, can get caught up in the mix of coping strategies here.

If you had your needs met, received care and attention and grew up with things around you feeling calmer and more stable, your brain will have had the opportunity to develop in a more balanced way. Although, do know that all of us are likely to experience some challenges or a degree of trauma in some shape or form — none of

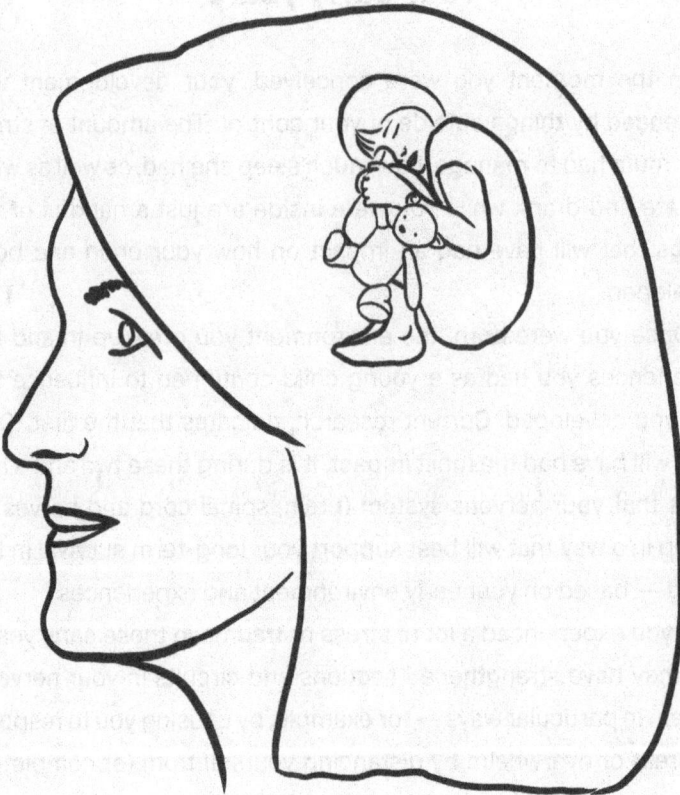

us escapes completely. We all have reasons to find a way to cope; it's just that some wounds are deeper than others.

In a nutshell, how your life was during your early years will likely be influencing some of your behaviours today.

————

Beyond your first two and a half years, your brain continued to adapt based on the information it received and processed from the culture you grew up in, your living environment, the people around you and the experiences you had. A huge part of what will have influenced the way you eat, your relationship with food, how you feel about your body and how you feel about yourself is the place and the people in your day-to-day living environment as a child.

If, like me, you grew up in a household where someone else was seemingly always on a diet or fixated on food, be it theirs or what *you* ate, this will have rubbed off on you. It will have affected your beliefs and the way you now think and feel about food and your body.

If money was tight at home, and food was never to be wasted and every last scrap eaten, this will likely be a pattern that replays in your life — because, deep down, you might believe that one day there won't be enough food again. And this is so even if the reality of your life right now is very different. The old belief can still be strong.

And what about your body? Was this commented on at home? Were you compared with a slimmer sibling? Did your brother or sister call you chubby? Were you told that you ate too much or your clothes were too tight, so you needed to eat less?

If you moved around from house to house within your extended family and had different food rules and eating patterns in each place, such as structured meals in one place and chaotic, irregular eating patterns in another, how did this make you feel and affect the way you think?

While working on this book, I asked on social media how my followers' eating habits had been influenced by their upbringing. The answers brought me to tears, and I know the same might be true for you. **So please know you are not alone.**

Here are some of those answers:

- 'I watched my mum yo-yo diet and was always told to pull my stomach in.'
- 'My mum weighed herself every day and complained about the number being too high, so I started weighing myself and always have that same thought now.'
- 'I was always given chocolate or sweets when I was upset and now do the same as an adult.'
- 'My dad told me I was getting too fat and to eat less.'
- 'I always had to finish my plate even if I wasn't hungry.'
- 'I was put on my first diet at 11 years old and at 42 I am only just trying to stop dieting.'
- 'My family always used to comment on what I ate, so now I don't like to eat in front of others.'
- 'We always had lots of sugary snacks at home growing up, I now find I do the same as it feels normal to have them in the house.'
- 'My family always commented on other people's bodies in front of me, saying they were too skinny or too fat.'
- 'My mum took me to a gym to lose weight when I was at primary school.'
- 'At 10 I was told my legs were fat and this has haunted me ever since.'
- 'I always felt like the fattest in our family, the shame was and still is so bad.'
- 'I was told not to eat after school because I was getting fat.'

TIME TO REFLECT: To get to understand yourself better, I highly recommend that you sit down in a quiet place for at least half an hour and just write about the history of your relationship with food and your body.

Here are some thought starters to reflect on as you go through this process:

- Was there always enough food to go around when you were younger? Did you feel like there was competition with your siblings or others you lived with to get enough food? Could it be that, even now, you still hold a belief that there isn't going to be enough food, even though in reality there is?
- Did you have to 'finish' everything on your plate? Do you still do this now?
- Did anyone ever comment on the shape and size of your body? How did that make you feel? How do you feel about your body now?
- Were your meals predictable or erratic? Do you now have a structure or an ad hoc way of eating?
- Were you often compared with another person, either in your household or out? What did you do when this happened? Eat more? Shut down? Get angry? What happens now when you are compared with others?
- Did anyone tell you to eat more, or eat less, or comment on how much food you ate? How do you feel now when someone comments on your eating?
- Was anyone in the house on a diet when you were growing up? Has this influenced how you think and behave around food now, do you think?
- Did you learn how to cook? Has this impacted how you eat now? Are your cooking skills a barrier to you eating the way you would like to eat?

There are so many questions I could ask you here, but the key thing is to think about how your current eating patterns, and how you think and feel about yourself now, might have been influenced by your living situation when you were younger.

Aim to approach this activity from a place of curiosity, rather than judgement on either yourself or others. It is not intended to encourage you to start sending unkind messages to your brother for stealing your food, or confront a relative about the comments they used to make about your thighs. Instead, it aims to help you understand *you*, and to see that part of the way you are is based on what you have been through.

I know that some of this might be hard to face, hard to think about and upsetting to reflect on. I wish I could take away some of the things that have been said to you or happened to you; but sadly, I don't have that magic power. However, I can help you stop these things ruling your life anymore.

This reflection will come in handy when we get to Chapter 5 and start looking at reprogramming your relationship with food.

My own reflection

When I was growing up, we were lucky enough to have enough to eat at home, although I was very aware that my mum's family hadn't always when she was a child, so that did play on my mind. Because of this I was very aware that food was not to be wasted, and I am pretty sure we had to finish most things on our plate.

Having two brothers, there was inherently what felt like a fight for food — but only because they ate so much and at a much faster pace than me! Sometimes there was none of my favourite cereal, no crumpets and none of the yoghurt I liked left because they had scoffed the lot. They never commented on my weight, as far as I remember, but they did certainly comment on what I ate.

We always ate our meals at the table — snacking wasn't really a thing in our house or at school. After breakfast at home we had milk mid-morning at school, and a hot cooked meal there at lunchtime, and then waited for dinner until we got home. At the weekend and the holidays, we went out on our bikes and were told to come home when it was getting dark, as that would mean it was dinnertime. So different to now, when it seems kids want to eat every hour and can't go anywhere without a stash of muesli bars or other such nibbles 'in case' the worst might happen and hunger strikes!

While my family didn't comment on my body until I lost weight, I remember always being conscious of my thighs, probably because my mum was so conscious of hers. She refused to wear swimming togs or shorts unless absolutely necessary. I guess off the back of this I learnt that your legs were something you could be ashamed of.

As I mentioned earlier, my mum also always used to 'body check' constantly — squeeze her legs, arms and stomach to see how much fat was on them. It was a habit I picked up — and have mostly learnt to curb, but not always. This is something that replays for me as an adult and I have had to work to address.

Beyond the younger years

The living situations and circumstances you experienced as you continued to grow up have also played their part in influencing your eating and drinking behaviours, your habits, and also how you feel about both your body and yourself.

When I moved out of home and lived in halls of residence at university, this threw things up in the air for me and my eating. After 14 years of being vegetarian, one night I had a few too many drinks and some leftover chicken curry and decided it was too hard to be vegetarian while I was flatting. So I started to eat meat again. I also started drinking a lot, as it was so built into uni culture and all the activities we did. From sports team pub crawls to 50-pence vodka shots on different nights of the week at the clubs in town, it became normal to drink way too much.

As for so many others, my eating changed dramatically in my first year of studying. With our flat-share food situation I started snacking more, eating a lot more chips, biscuits and fried food; things I had never really had much of before. My body changed a lot, which wasn't helped by the fact that on top of the unbalanced eating I was still bingeing at that time.

Flatting with dietitians in my second, third and fourth years did help a bit, because at least our meals were more balanced, but the hard drinking carried on and my own eating issues of bingeing, vomiting and laxative abuse remained rife.

Not long after university, I moved to New Zealand and started flatting with people who had an interest in health and wellbeing — which meant more veg, nourishing snacks, slightly less booze, plenty of walks and gym time! It is a lot easier to make healthier choices when the people around you are on the same wavelength as you and have a vision that is aligned with your goals.

From flatting, I moved in with my now-husband and had to navigate around the way *he* was eating. As a gym buff at the time, he was committed to grilled chicken, broccoli, protein shakes and supplements and didn't have anywhere near enough variety in his food. At first his control around food was a big trigger for me, as I was coming out the other end of my bulimic journey and working to be less controlled with my eating, but over time he managed to be more flexible with his eating, too.

Now, in my current phase of life with two children and juggling that with working full-time, my eating habits and behaviours have changed yet again. The types of food we eat are slightly different to pre-children, and a lot more snacking happens because, with being so active, my kids need to eat a couple more times a day than I do. When life is full-on and you are driving back and forth from activity to activity after school so mealtimes aren't consistent, it can be a real challenge to eat in a way that is helpful and works for your body. I had to find ways to adapt, which includes meal planning, cooking in bulk and having quick and easy meal options at the ready.

Given my studies and interests, I know I have been lucky with my living situations, and I have actively made choices in my older years to live with people who support a balanced way of eating. Of course, it might not be the same for you. I know it is hard to live with people whose food goals don't align with yours or who have food issues that clash with yours.

TIME TO REFLECT: Have a think about how other people in and around your living situation may have influenced your eating behaviour. Write notes if it is helpful. Here are a few questions which might help get you started, but don't be limited by these — there are so many other things that may be in the mix, too!

- Have you lived at any time with someone who significantly impacted the way you eat in an unhelpful way? For example, did you feel judged by someone else when you were eating in front of them?
- Do you have a partner, flatmate or friend who often brings you treats or takeaways, or makes rich, delicious meals, so you end up eating more than you want to or eating things you would really rather not?
- If you live on your own, do you struggle to be motivated to eat well or cook? Or do you eat to feel less lonely?
- Do your cooking facilities or time pressures limit or impact your choices when it comes to food and what you can practically prepare, both for yourself and for others?

The people around you

Beyond the influence of your living environment comes the powerful nature of the other people in your orbit as you move through life.

The friends you have made, and those you have lost. The people you connect with socially, some who you feel like you have known for years after one night out, and others who you see over and over again at the school gates or sideline of the sports field but never really gel with.

From the learning phases of life, your teachers, lecturers, mentors and the friends (and foes) you had at school, college or university.

The people you have dated, the ones who have had crushes on you, and the ones you wanted to date but never felt brave enough to ask. The ones who broke your heart or broke your trust.

Your partners, ex-partners, spouses, ex-spouses, soon-to-be ex-spouses, or — often the most complex of all — your ex-spouse's new partner. Ouch, that one often hurts.

And what about people connected with events, sports, clubs, activities, be it out or online? Or the people who you work with, have worked with, or worked for. Your colleagues, your bosses, your peers . . . and that lady in the office who you always feel is judging you no matter *what* you do.

The people we interact with throughout our lives change us. Their words, reactions, responses, facial expressions and body language can all influence how we think and feel about ourselves and, as a result, how we behave. From a random comment from a stranger which stays in your head, to the way your boss looked at you in a meeting about restructuring the business, to a friend's overly direct comment when she'd had too much to drink — we make these interactions mean something. And they change us because, to varying degrees, we care about what other people think. Humans are social beings, and being accepted by others is part of what helps us feel safe. Feeling like you are part of a group, a tribe or a team matters; and when it doesn't work out that way, it doesn't feel good.

TIME TO REFLECT: Have a think, now and over the coming days, about this question: How have other people you have interacted with in your life affected how you think, how you feel about yourself and how you behave?

Again . . . ditch the judgement and blame here. Look for the lessons in this.

Social media

Back when I was growing up, it was the images of Kylie Minogue on her newest music cassette, the late Olivia Newton-John playing Sandy in the movie *Grease* and other images appearing in magazines that had the biggest impact on my friends and me and how we thought we should look. And that was: slim, toned, and stereo-typically 'pretty' based on what was seen to be ideal in those days.

But while diet books were rife, leotards were tight and the WeightWatchers brand was everywhere, it was much easier to escape body comparisons and diet culture messages than it is today. With the rise of social media, filtered photos and videos as well as those that are AI-generated, every minute of every day at the touch of a button we are thrust into a world of content that we can compare ourselves against. At the time of writing, it is estimated that there are 6.9 billion images per day shared on WhatsApp, 3.8 billion images per day posted on Snapchat, 2.1 billion on Facebook and 1.3 billion on Instagram. On those four platforms alone, that is nearly 164,000 per second!!

The images we compare ourselves with are so often not a reflection of reality, which can be both tragic and dangerous. Even if you don't add a filter to your photos on an app, to some degree the camera on your phone is still doing it for you anyway. I remember taking a photo of the stretch marks on my legs, which are really pronounced, to share how normal it is to have scars and marks on your body — but when I went to review the photo, the marks had been softened and were far less obvious than in real life. My camera phone had automatically changed them to make it a 'better photo'. But that better photo became a lie about what was real.

The more you search on a particular topic, the more images and content of a similar type you will be served up by the algorithms behind these platforms, which are acting like an echo chamber. Then there are Facebook groups, communities and chat rooms you can join which further reinforce the same messages. I once searched on 'thigh gap' for an article I was writing about body dysmorphia, as I kept hearing people talk about their goal being to lose enough weight or do the right workouts to get a visible gap between their tights when they stood with their legs together. For weeks afterwards I got content and ads sharing the latest tips and tricks for reducing inner thigh fat and getting a gap. Please, do not put 'thigh gap' in your search box.

While I try my very best to post unfiltered real-life images of myself, I fully admit that I don't look like I look on social media all the time — especially at 5 a.m. after being woken up by kids multiple times throughout the night! My life isn't exactly what you see, either. I remember the other day posting a photo of my team and me going out for lunch at an annual get-together where I genuinely had a wonderful time and my smile in the photos was 100% real; but beyond those hours together, things were not that great at all. My dad, who has cancer, was unwell, and I was worried about him.

A family friend had died a few days before from the same cancer my dad has. My husband and I were at a standoff about what felt like everything, from where we live to our hours of work and how to manage the kids. My son was having some issues at school which I knew I needed to address urgently. I was in the middle of the launch of a new online platform and we were having some technical problems. Then our water pump broke, meaning no drinking water, showers, flushing toilet or washing machine.

You could see none of this behind the smiling photo of me at lunch. It wasn't that I was intentionally hiding any of those issues, but more that I was in the middle of processing it all and wanted to enjoy being present with my team despite all the stuff going on.

No one can share every minute of their life online — and nor should they, to be honest — but there is something we all need to be highly aware of as we scroll through our feed. **The moments you see are a snapshot, not a full reflection of reality.**

TIME TO REFLECT: Have a good think about how much you are being influenced by who you follow on social media, in terms of how their content and messages are impacting the way you eat and drink as well as how you think and feel about yourself.

- Are the people you are following helping you genuinely take steps in a positive direction, making you laugh or feel inspired?
- Or are they motivating you by the feeling of shame? Are some people you follow actually making you feel bad about yourself, and like you aren't doing enough and not getting your nutrition or training 'right'?

Even when your best friend or a trusted colleague at work recommends that you follow someone because their approach works for them, it does not mean that this will necessarily be right for you. You need to be selective.

I cannot recommend a social media declutter highly enough. A few years ago I stopped following all other nutritionists and dietitians because it was just making me feel like I wasn't doing enough. Their ideas all seemed better than mine, I didn't have the online programmes they did, and I wasn't posting recipes that looked as good as theirs. Following them also made me feel like maybe I needed to be more restrictive with my own diet, because even credible people who I was following were at times suggesting measuring and weighing food out, which for me would have been a big step in the wrong direction based on my history. Having their views and opinions in my face every day took me away from doing my best, authentic work, made me doubt myself and only pushed me towards unhelpful coping strategies to numb the difficult emotions, which for me were ice cream or alcohol.

Book in your unfollowing session — it is time for a declutter!

The 'health' industry

There is a need for an industry that supports us to be healthier, to optimise our wellbeing and enjoy our lives. I am part of that industry, and there is some phenomenal work done by many in this space. However, as in most industries, there are cowboys. Businesses large and small with immoral groundings who are consciously willing to exploit people's weaknesses to financially benefit from their pain, fears and worries.

These businesses have encouraged us to judge our bodies for their differences or perceived 'flaws'. They have helped shape the belief that fat is to be feared, that a larger body is not as desirable as a smaller one, and that if you have dewy-looking skin and less cellulite then your life will somehow be better.

The food industry is tied up in the mix here. From one food trend to another, along with the clever packaging and the confusing market-ing claims, it is a minefield to work out what is a healthy choice for you and what's not. Businesses are there to make money first and foremost, so don't be fooled into believing that in some way, deep down, they really care about what's best for you — only a handful of businesses really do. Even some pharmacies, often seen as trusted places to get advice, can get caught up in the action. Some of the large-scale chains, and a handful of the smaller ones, are essentially endorsing diet-culture messages with their regular promotion of meal replacement shakes and weight-loss supplements.

There is so much money to be made from these promises to solve our insecurities, and you have no doubt paid into that pot at some point. The global weight-loss and diet industry was estimated to be worth US$280 billion in 2024, predicted to rise to US$471 billion in 2029. This is an industry that isn't going anywhere fast, which is a tragedy — not only because the spending is often ineffective, with around two-thirds of people ending up regaining the weight they lost through dieting practices, but also because the process of dieting erodes people's self-worth.

Along with social media and advertising, the diet industry has also fuelled the rate of dieting and disordered eating. The other day, just before the news came on, there was an advert for a 'man shake' on TV: a meal replacement shake that promised 'weight loss made easy' with those classic 'before' and 'after' photos at the forefront of the promotion. This sparked my seven-year-old to ask: 'Dad, do you need the man shakes to get your six-pack back?' This then turned into both my boys having a conversation about needing to have a six-pack like Batman, and holding up their T-shirts to see how many 'packs' they had. My seven-year-old said three. (I was quite pleased that on this occasion he didn't know how to count abs properly.)

As well as the cowboys, there are those who can unintentionally cause harm in this industry, a result of either lack of awareness or lack of training.

Laura, a friend of mine in the UK, recently had to take her daughter to the doctor to get a prescription for antibiotics. As part of the process, her daughter had to be weighed so they could get the dose of the medication right. On their way home, Laura's daughter turned to her and asked, 'Is there something wrong with my weight and height?'

Of course, Laura said no, not at all. Then, puzzled, she asked her daughter why she thought that. And the reply was that the way the nurse looked at her and a comment she made about her weight as she stepped off the scales made her feel like there was something wrong with her and the numbers. Did this maybe mean she was too heavy? Too short? Or too tall?

While weighing may have been necessary in this case, to establish the correct drug dosage, the comments and judgement weren't. It is interactions like this where big problems can start.

There is a reason why at my wellbeing practice Mission Nutrition we don't weigh our clients unless (very occasionally) there is a justifiable clinical reason to do so. We are there to help our clients improve the way they eat, how they think and feel about themselves, and their overall wellbeing — not define their success and self-worth by a number on the scales.

If you have been on the diet rollercoaster before, feel like you can't trust yourself around food, don't have the willpower it takes to get results, or need to have lists of rules to be 'healthy', then please know: **you are not the problem**. This mixed-up industry full of false promises and conflicting information is the problem. Set alongside our environment which supports and encourages drinking, overconsumption, upsizing and sweet treats to 'cheer you up' after a hard day, it is no wonder that so many of us are in such a pickle when it comes to the way we eat and how we feel about our bodies and ourselves.

Give yourself a break for the false starts, past attempts and the energy you have wasted. Let's put that journey behind you and move forward with a more compassionate approach right now.

Beauty standards

Part of your foundations relating to how you think and feel about your body, and how much and what types of foods you feel you 'should' eat, will be based on what was considered 'ideal' or 'desirable' in the culture you grew up in, as well as the views in the places where you have lived throughout your life.

Where my brother lives in France, it's seen as pretty abnormal to be in a larger body unless you are in your older years. It is also normal to eat your veges first and to make food from scratch, and taking a break for lunch is an absolute must.

In the Pacific Islands, a bigger body is considered beautiful, and curviness is often celebrated. Food is love, and if your friends and family leave your house feeling hungry then there must be a problem.

In Japan, being slim and having pale skin is viewed as optimal. When I was in Japan, I also noticed that food was something to be respected, snacking was a rarity, and eating on the go was nowhere near as common as it is over here. Sitting down and committing to eating at mealtimes seemed to be the norm.

In Brazil, as my Brazilian friends often remind me, it's important to try to look good. That means putting make-up on regardless of whether you are going to school pick-up, the supermarket or a big night out, and always making sure that your nails look tidy and your hair is in place.

On my last trip to the UK I noticed that, as in many other countries, the flavour of the moment seems to be a bigger bum that looks like you love squats, plumped-up lips and a tanned glow whatever the weather.

And as for here, on this side of the world in New Zealand and Australia, despite messages around body shape and size slowly becoming more balanced and with a marginally increased acceptance of variety, the ideal still commonly recognised is being slim but not too thin, a flat stomach, no wobbles on your arms and no visible cellulite, as well as being toned but not too muscly. It is a hard game to win!

In recent years, in addition to the shape and size of our bodies being judged, how our skin, make-up and hair look now seems to be more important than ever. Glossy hair, make-up that makes you look naturally flawless and as though you have no make-up on (but took half an hour to do), and fewer wrinkles are on many a wish-list. Ageing gracefully is also on that list, and with that comes the expensive creams, collagen products and shampoo recommendations.

These are generalisations, of course, and things do vary massively from one place to another; but the overall message is that in some way, shape or form, how we look and the size of our bodies is something that in many cultures seems to really matter. The result is that we both consciously and unconsciously judge ourselves for the way we look, and commonly feel the need to change ourselves to try and 'fit in' to the norm.

Being aware of what is influencing us is the first step to being able to make our own choices about the messages we are willing to buy into and those we choose to let go of.

TIME TO REFLECT: Have a think about what messages you got about your body when you were growing up. Do you still hold on to any food rules from your childhood which no longer help you? Later in the book when we come to reprogramming your eating behaviour, some of your reflections here might come in handy, so make notes if you like.

Our food environment

If you reflect on the types and variety of food you had access to growing up, it is likely to be different to now. With fast-food outlets here, there and everywhere, supermarkets open 24/7 in some places, and everything from petrol stations to airports offering an array of tasty treats at all hours of the day and night, it has become increasingly easy and normal to eat foods we never used to far more often than is healthy for our bodies and minds.

I believe, and research backs this up, that our food environment is one of the biggest influences on the way we eat. As a nation, if we want to support ourselves in making more nourishing food choices more often, our food environment needs a dramatic make-over.

At the end of the day — regardless of what you know about nutrition and wellbeing — if you are busy and time-poor, you often end up defaulting to the easiest, most accessible option. Sure, it is super-helpful to be able to pick up groceries at 3 a.m. if you are a shift worker, or sometimes grab a sandwich on the go, but having a doughnut stand open at 6 a.m. before early-morning flights at the airport? Really?

When you are making choices about what to buy, particularly given the crazy cost of living these days, you are also likely to be highly swayed by price and what seems the 'best value', even though sometimes this encourages you to actually spend more and eat/drink more than your body really needs. Take the example of a popular smoothie chain offering small, medium and large drinks. The small one, sitting at 225 ml, is $6.90. The medium one, 400 ml, is $9, so for only $2.10 more you get almost double the volume — so it seems logical to upsize, right?

What about the large one, at 500 ml and $9.60? For just an extra 60 cents you get 100 ml more than the medium! This makes it by far the most cost-effective option. Pricing the drinks this way can push you to buy nearly twice the amount of smoothie for only an extra $2.70, which seems like a bargain. But in reality you actually spent nearly $3 more, probably had a drink that was far bigger than you actually wanted, and at the same time upsized from 10 teaspoons to 19 teaspoons of sugar.

Going back to my example of doughnuts at the airport, when you buy a six-pack of these you essentially get one free compared with the cost of buying them singly. From my very frequent trips to the airport, I have seen that this is a very popular option even first thing in the morning.

Please don't underestimate how much you are being influenced by the power of marketing and pricing models that encourage you to upsize. They are invisible influences which could have a massive impact on your eating and drinking behaviour.

Don't get me wrong: I am not saying 'Never eat doughnuts, burgers or smoothies'. I'm simply asking you to be aware that easy access to foods like this, along with the bright shop lights, the smells and the special offers, are encouraging you to make choices that are often not likely to have been either intentional or mindfully influenced.

And while I am all for personal responsibility in many aspects of life, this is one place where I fundamentally disagree with that concept. Thinking that either we or our children should easily be able to avoid the lure of readily available, in-our-faces, manipulative marketing and the like which plays into our psychological weaknesses and leads us into choices which sabotage our intentions is so unhelpful. *Massive* amounts of money, time and resources are put into exploiting aspects of our behaviour. **It is just wrong that we should be made to feel like we are the ones who can't control ourselves** when we live in a world where these forces are at play, manipulating us in such crafty ways.

Beyond the influence of food companies, the availability and accessibility of food to children in our schools and to us in our places of work can also be huge. I have done a massive amount of work with both large and small businesses over the years to support them to improve the health and wellbeing of their staff, and one of the most important places to start is by looking at the food and drink options available in the workplace. Far too many businesses had lolly jars, cookie tins, fridges full of alcohol, and large coffee machines without offering any healthier alternatives or making it easier for staff to prepare and eat more nourishing options. Yes, there should be choices for all, but if we want to be able to feel good and function well, it really needs to be much easier for all of us to make choices that support our wellbeing. When so much of our eating is habitual, this is just common sense.

TIME TO REFLECT: How much does your current food environment at home, work and in the places you visit regularly influence your eating and drinking behaviour? Do you get lured into buying specials and upsizing?

Ideas of success

Beyond all of those many messages about what an ideal body needs to look like, there are also messages we absorb about what it means to have a successful life or to feel like you are 'good enough'. This, too, varies from culture to culture, but is commonly defined by things like how much money you earn, your job title, your status in the community, the car you drive, whether you are in a relationship and whether you have had children or not.

It is easy to get caught up trying to build a life chasing ideals of success that might tick someone else's box of acceptance but don't create any internal fulfilment or joy for us; or, worse still, create a sense of disconnect from who we feel we really are.

I am lucky enough to have been brought up with what feels to me like a wholesome ideal of what success is. My family judges success on creating a life that is meaningful where you make a positive impact on the world and the people around you, which is what I chase and my dream. I appreciate, however, that not everyone had the same luck as me in this space.

TIME TO REFLECT: But what about you? Growing up, how was success defined to you? How, do you think, has this impacted the choices you now make?

If you are currently living a life that feels like it isn't the success you would like, or you have all the success you dreamed of and more but feel empty, then you aren't broken! This situation is most likely because you are not correctly aligned with who you are and what really matters to you. We will be exploring this in Chapters 11 and 12.

Part 2

Learning to re-think your relationship with food

Chapter 3
The role food plays in our lives

At its most basic level, food is essential for our survival, because it provides the energy and nutrients our bodies need to function. Beyond that, however, food plays many other roles in our lives, offering enrichment in so many ways.

Yesterday, on my way back from doing a radio interview in the city, I popped into my aunty and uncle's house for a cuppa and a catch-up. One cup turned into another, and while sipping our tea we shared stories about road trips, weddings, work, friends and adventures we had planned. When dinnertime rolled around, our chats were still going strong. A bottle of red was opened and I stayed and enjoyed the most delicious fish pie I've ever had.

As we sat and enjoyed the food and wine, we talked about where the fish had come from, the cost of different types of seafood and the fun my aunty and uncle had had at the fish market that day. We then reminisced about times we had been fishing together, before sharing stories of the broken tractor we used to use to get their tin boat to the beach, and how fun it was making tuatua fritters together many moons ago.

Eating can bring us together. Sharing food is a wonderful opportunity to connect with friends, family or strangers, sharing stories, ideas and world-views. Be it an evening meal with the people you live with or fish and chips on the beach after a day in the water, this shared experience can help you feel closer to people.

Food can also hold profound psychological significance. Certain foods evoke memories and emotions, triggering feelings of nostalgia and comfort. From the aroma of freshly baked bread to the taste of a favourite meal from childhood, be it your grandma's lasagne or your mum's choc-chip cookies, food has the amazing power of transporting us through time and space in the most incredible way.

There are many celebrations that also centre around food and drink. When I last went home to the UK, I was there for Christmas. As well as enjoying all the festive lights, Christmas carols and embracing the cold, we spent a huge amount of time planning and preparing foods that are part of our family traditions.

First up is sorting the turkey, which we always get from our local butcher, Dean. He's so popular that you have to get up at the crack of dawn and get into line well before the shop opens. If you don't, you'll be there for at least two hours, in the cold, waiting to get in, with the queue going around the block! This trip to the butcher and chatting with other customers in the line about their Christmas plans is a yearly tradition that feels like part of the celebration.

Next comes prepping my mum's super-special roast potatoes, which means hunting down the specific type of potatoes that work best. This sometimes involves trips to a couple of different shops because crispy spuds are a vital part of the festive lunch. The final part of preparations, on Christmas Eve, involves trying to get as much brandy into the brandy butter as humanly possible. This requires getting the butter to the right temperature, whipping it correctly, and making sure not to do this too early or it will separate — a Christmas Day disaster!

While Christmas isn't celebrated by everyone, in all our cultures there are celebrations where food plays a central role. You will no doubt be able to think of some ways in which food and drinks are intertwined with your culture and the things you celebrate.

Making food is also something that some people really enjoy. Cooking can be a fantastic creative outlet, an opportunity to try new things, experiment with flavours and develop new skills as you go. When I have the time, I love nothing more than trying out new recipes and ideas. Sometimes I come up with masterpieces which go down a treat, although often I can't re-create a dish because my approach to cooking is a creative 'add a bit of this and a bit of that and see how it works out'. But even when my creations aren't such a win, I still enjoy the process. I realise that this isn't true for everyone. I have friends who would rather eat spiders than get into creative 'throw together' cooking.

Last, but not least, food can be really delicious. Enjoying food that tastes good has got to be one of life's most incredible pleasures. From new-season apples and a ripe avocado to crispy dumplings and a flavour-packed green curry, eating tasty food can make you feel good. Really good!

The flip side of food being intertwined with so many things we do is that it can be easy to eat when we don't really need or want to eat. As I mentioned earlier in the book, I call this unhelpful eating behaviour because if you find that this happens regularly, it can sabotage your wellbeing goals. You could end up struggling with low energy, your clothes not fitting you anymore, developing a health condition related to eating more than your body needs, or just generally not feeling so good about yourself.

The same goes for alcohol. While a glass of wine at the weekend with your friends over dinner is one thing, drinking every night to manage stress is quite another. With the myriad negative effects that too much alcohol can cause on both your body and your mind, that certainly can become a problem.

───────

When it comes to a healthy relationship with food, there is absolutely no 'one size fits all' definition. There are many different thoughts, opinions and experiences with food that will play into what ends up being defined as a 'healthy relationship' with food. But here is where I sit: I believe that **having a healthy relationship with food means that when you eat you feel good about it before, during and afterwards, most of the time**.

To be able to get to this place, you need the ability to mindfully and intentionally make informed choices about what you eat, based on the best outcomes for you and the goals in your life. Your goals might include things like supporting your body to work at its best, having enough energy to do the things you enjoy, or maintaining a healthy immune system so you aren't always sick and run-down.

This also means being able to make intentional choices about enjoying things like the odd slice of cake, packet of salt and vinegar chips, or a pie on the mountain after skiing because, in balance, **all foods can all be part of a healthy, fulfilling life**. Equally, however, it means being able to say 'no thanks' to the free cookie on the plane if you don't really want it, or to a second serving of breakfast at an all-you-can-eat hotel buffet because you aren't hungry enough and really know that your body doesn't want more food at this time.

The key words to tune in to here are **mindfully** and **intentionally**, which I talked about on pages 30–31. If you decide, and you feel good about your choice (most of the time!), you are on to a win, and this is what I would refer to as helpful eating behaviour. The reality is, however, that for so many of us much of the eating we do is mindless. This means that often our choices are based on what is easiest to access, quickest to eat and fills a gap (be that hunger or an emotional hole) — and that is unhelpful eating behaviour.

The good news is that with awareness and practice, you can re-program your eating to be more mindful and intentional; plus, by managing your environment you can make it much easier to make food choices that make you feel good before, during and after eating. Coming up, I will explain exactly how to do that so that you can be back in the driver's seat of your choices without any need for obsession, hyperfocus or restriction.

I also believe that having a healthy relationship with food means that **most of the time** you eat in tune with your body's natural inbuilt hunger and fullness signals. That means eating when you are hungry and stopping eating when you are full.

Like I said, though, this is *most* of the time — it doesn't mean 100% of the time. There are always exceptions, like the piece of pizza I ate yesterday when my friends ordered some after the kids' sports game. I wasn't really that hungry, but *man* it looked good. So I ate it, enjoyed it and moved on, because this is not what I do most of the time.

If you have dieted for years, or always followed a 'plan', I know that hunger and fullness signals might not be something you feel like you know anymore. But they *are* something you can get back in tune with. I will be talking about this more in Chapter 4.

Lastly, having a healthy relationship with food, in my view, means **there is no guilt associated with eating,** or drinking for that matter. Having guilt around food serves no purpose other than robbing you of joy and making you feel disappointed with yourself, so let's park it. Thinking about what you 'should eat', what you did eat and running through your mind all the things you could have done differently is soul-destroying. I know. I did it for much of my life.

It is time to let this judgement go.

Chapter 4

Getting back in tune with your body

I t is now time to crack into the 'action' part of this book, where I help you take some positive steps in the right direction to help you improve your relationship with food and with yourself. This includes giving yourself permission to eat, getting back in tune with your body by understanding hunger and fullness, as well as practising mindful eating.

I will then help you understand what's not working for you, before (in Chapter 5) taking you through my four-step process that will help you rewire any deeply embedded unhelpful eating patterns you have.

———

As a nutritionist, one of the things I get asked *all* the time is 'How much should I eat?' While there are guidelines and recommendations for an overall framework (which I will take you through in Chapter 8) and this can be helpful as a starting point, it is also really important to know that **the amount you need to eat every day can vary**. There will be some days when you will feel hungrier than others; in winter you are likely to want more than in summer, due to the weather — and that is all within the realms of very normal. Aiming to eat to a plan that is too prescriptive is really unhelpful and can mess with your mind — something you have no doubt done a million times before, and possibly why you chose this book over yet another 'diet-focused' one.

This is why at Mission Nutrition we are loath to give strict meal plans, and it is also why in this book I am not going to tell you exactly what to eat in a day with cups of this and grams of that. Instead, my mission is to help you understand the **key principles** so you can make choices that help you feel good and your body to work at its best, while also ensuring you know that flexibility and **finding what works for you and your body is paramount**. You might find that fewer carbs works for you but not for your friend, even if she is the same age and at the same stage as you. You might also find that more protein at dinner is what *you* need, but with *her* daily routine a really solid protein-packed breakfast and less protein at dinner is required.

I know that to some degree it is helpful to know what to do — it helps you plan and get into a routine — but at any given time when you eat, the amount you need to eat must be based on how *you* feel and what is right for *you*.

This is something you might need to relearn how to do.

When you were born, without logical thought you knew you had to cry when you needed food, and you were able to stop feeding when you had had enough. We arrive in the world with the ability to regulate the amount we eat, but 'food rules', our unhelpful food environment, our busy lives and our easy access to foods that make it hard to stop eating have all made accessing this inbuilt process more challenging. If you were ever encouraged to finish what was on your plate, or told you couldn't have seconds because you were putting on weight, or found yourself eating a handful more chips than you planned to, you will know exactly what I mean.

There is good news, though! This intuitive ability is still accessible to you, and it can be retrained by saying goodbye to restrictive diets and getting back in tune with your body's signals.

Permission to eat

If dieting or some form of food restriction has been part of your journey so far or is something you are doing right now, then giving yourself **permission to eat enough food each day** is something you will need to work on as you go through the reprogramming process.

You shouldn't feel like you need to eat like a little bird, be totally sugar/carb/refined food free or follow a list of strict 'rules' to be healthy. Because this isn't healthy. It's obsessional and a story that has been created by diet culture or people on the internet trying to sell you things or scare you into action. Quite honestly, it is just not okay for people to use fear in their messaging.

We would (or should) never take an extreme restrictive approach to our children's nutrition, so why do we think it is okay to do it to ourselves? Not feeding yourself enough food often means diving head-first into a box of cereal at 10 p.m., or picking at the leftover dinner you didn't let yourself have enough of just before you go to bed. Also, banishing lengthy lists of foods from your list of options often only leads to you wanting them more. Restriction can often lead to overeating and feeling out of control with food, like you just can't stop when you finally 'give in' to the foods you have been trying so hard to avoid. The restrict–binge cycle is a common one, and it really messes with your mind. This is no way to live. You shouldn't have to have a rule that makes you feel like you've sinned when you haven't been able to follow it!

Following restrictive patterns of eating for too long can cause huge amounts of stress and anxiety, too. When you are constantly thinking of what you are going to be eating, how you might manage social situations, and contemplating whether some events are just best avoided because of the food, it really can steal the joy from your life.

Restriction can also become an addiction in its own right, and can end up becoming an eating disorder if followed to the extreme. When what you are eating — or trying not to eat — becomes a key focus of your life, it can be incredibly destructive. I know. I've been there and it's somewhere I wouldn't want to be again.

It is important to note the **context** in which I am talking about restriction in this book. There are times when there might be foods you are best to moderate or remove from your diet — if, for example, you are pregnant, or you have diagnosed allergies or intolerances, or you're managing things like IBS (irritable bowel syndrome), and you are being advised by a qualified health professional who knows your personal medical history and needs. It's quite a different thing to have a list of 'banned' or 'bad' foods based on a desire to change your weight or body size, or because a 'guru' on Instagram or a YouTube link your friend sent you told you to because otherwise you will die young. This second type of restriction is the type I am addressing here. The type that involves limiting your food, obsessively tracking or counting it so that it takes over your entire head-space and makes you feel anxious. Or following lists of 'rules' based on things that are 'good' or 'bad' for you without taking into account the bigger picture — nutrition that helps your body work well.

Letting go of restriction and leaning into permission

If you are currently restricting what you eat or following some strict food rules, I really do know that giving yourself permission to eat can be scary. Especially if you have been restricting your eating for a while — there is comfort in what is familiar. I had regularly restricted my food and ignored my body's hunger signals for over 15 years by the time I came to the realisation that something needed to change. When I reached the point where I knew I simply *had* to address my restriction, because I could see how it was leading to my bingeing, it still felt like I was losing part of my identity.

Letting go of restriction isn't something you can change overnight, and nor it is something you can just will yourself to do. Like most things in this book, it is a process; a journey. But it is a journey that will lead to a better, healthier, happier place for you.

If this is something that resonates with you, the first step is to acknowledge that food restriction is a behaviour you have — but it is not who you are. Language matters here. 'I have a binge-eating behaviour' is very different from 'I am a binge eater'. It is important to separate yourself from the behaviour.

The second step is to consider the pros and cons of this behaviour — so you can see not only why you are doing it, but also what it is costing you. What are the downsides?

Note: if restricting has been an issue for you in the past but isn't at the moment, you might still want to look through the questions coming up to see if you can glean any insight into what has drawn you into dieting or restriction in the past. This might well help you avoid getting sucked in again.

TIME TO REFLECT: When you have a quiet few moments, think about these questions:

- What do you get out of restricting your eating at times? Do you love seeing the numbers go down on the scales? Do you feel too scared not to restrict? Do you feel like you are in control of something when you follow the 'rules'? Or is it something else?
- Is the restriction or following the 'rules' giving you a sense of belonging because you are doing this with others?
- Are you seeking approval from others when you make your eating choices?
- What else are you getting from being really strict and rigid with your eating?

There are no right or wrong answers here. Just see what comes up for you.

Next, think about what the downsides might be. What is it costing you to hold on to the need to restrict your food at times or to be really rigid with your eating? Reflect on these questions:

- Do you feel like you think about food all the time?
- Do you worry about what you are going to eat in different situations?
- Have you ever felt like avoiding social situations because of it being a challenge to manage your eating/drinking there?
- Do you feel like food controls you and you would be lost without some form of restriction?
- Do you feel guilty when you eat?
- Do you get angry with yourself when you aren't able to follow the 'rules' or the plan?

- Is how you eat having a negative impact on your relationships with other people? And, more importantly, yourself?

As you will see, there are lots of downsides. The cost of continuing to restrict your eating or being too rigid is high. When, instead, you grant yourself permission to eat, this is the beginning of the journey to break free from the guilt and shame associated with 'failing' to follow dieting rules. Giving yourself permission to eat allows you to choose foods based on what your body needs, knowing that, over time, your body has the ability to make balanced and nutritious choices naturally.

We need to eat to live, and we need to eat enough to be satisfied. We just need to have the right tools to manage *how* we eat, *when* we eat and *how much* we eat, and these tools are already inside us. We just need to reconnect with them.

Honouring hunger and fullness

Learning to recognise how your body and mind communicate with you, and to be able to honour the messages they send, can be one of the most powerful journeys you can go on to reconnect with yourself.

Hunger and **fullness** are two messages you can tune in to for help regulating the amount you eat — rather than relying on a list, the scales or a rigid plan as the decision-maker. These messages are sensations you experience which let you know when your body needs nourishment and when it's had enough. The messages are controlled by a complex system of physical and hormonal signals and involve many parts of your body, including your brain, nervous system and gut. **Ghrelin** and **leptin** are the two primary hormones involved, and they do some amazing things!

When you haven't eaten for a while, you start to feel hungry and you might experience a rumbling stomach, light-headedness and (if you are anything like my younger son) being 'hangry'! At this time your stomach and other parts of your gut are producing **ghrelin**, which increases your appetite and your gut motility (movement of food through your gut) and ramps up the amount of acid your stomach produces. Ghrelin is highest when your stomach is empty or your blood sugar levels are low, and can create that growling sensation that rolls around when your body is asking for food. How clever!

When you have eaten and your body has had enough, your fat cells secrete the hormone **leptin**, which interacts with your brain and communicates that no more food is needed, and it is time to stop eating. At the same time, your ghrelin decreases, further reducing your drive to eat more.

Hunger differs from **appetite**, which is simply the desire to eat. Appetite is sometimes driven by hunger, but it can also be activated by walking past a bakery that is wafting out smells of freshly baked bread and pastries or by the smell of something cooking. If you are genuinely hungry and were offered a carrot or plain crackers, you would likely want to eat them; but if you only fancy ice cream or chips, it might be that appetite rather than true hunger is driving your feelings of wanting to eat. This is one of the huge challenges with our current food environment, which aims to trigger people's appetite with smells, pictures and special offers that can make them feel like they need to eat even when they really don't.

The types of food you eat can have a big impact on your hunger and fullness levels. Those which are packed with fibre, protein and fat have the biggest impact. Highly processed foods that are high in sugar and salt as well as low in fibre, however, don't help you feel full for long because they dump sugar into your blood much more quickly, especially when eaten on their own.

There are other processes in our bodies that affect hunger and appetite, too.

Do you feel hungrier before your period? This is normal. The hormonal changes that occur with your body effectively gearing up for a potential pregnancy can affect both your appetite and also the types of food you feel like eating. I know how hard it can be when you might be feeling like you are in a really good routine, but then — after eating like you normally would — somehow mid-morning you are craving something sweet and then, just before bed, you are right into jam on toast or a big bowl of cereal because your desire for carbs is off the charts. Please know that it is normal to eat a bit more food at this time, and that focusing on getting plenty of fibre and protein can be really helpful to support satiety (that feeling of fullness).

Are you not sleeping well and craving more carbs the next day? This is also normal. Sleep, which I will be talking about in Chapter 7, has a huge impact on your appetite. When the amount of sleep you are getting is inadequate, your leptin drops and your ghrelin increases so you get a double-whammy effect — a drive to eat more alongside poorer signals to stop eating! So if this is happening to you, improving your sleep would be one of the first places to focus your attention as it can make such a big difference.

If you are sleep-deprived, you are also more likely to crave carb-rich, sugary and salty foods, which is so ridiculously unhelpful. There are many theories around why our bodies do this, with one of the most widely believed being that sleep deprivation leads to the brain communicating that the body is in some sort of danger — this may mean there is a threat of starvation ahead, so stocking up body stores is vital to increase the chances of survival. We are the only animal species that consistently and consciously deprives ourselves of sleep. Your brain cannot possibly realise that it is late-night Netflix or inbox management that is driving the sleep deprivation; it simply reacts in a way that it thinks is the best for us.

Sleep deprivation is a real challenge for shift workers, and if you are one then you will know this all too well. Shift work totally messes with your system, so adjusting your life to ensure you get enough sleep even when you're working unusual hours is key.

Exercise is another thing that can influence how hungry you feel. When you exercise, you commonly want to eat more food; but over time, for some people, exercise may reduce hunger. Appetite can also be increased with certain medications, which is something that happens with a medication I have to take, so I understand the challenges here. This is something to be aware of and to discuss with your doctor if you notice it happening to you. There may be other medication options for you to try.

The hunger and fullness scale

Becoming tuned in to the factors that are driving your eating, as well as how hungry you are before you start eating and how full you are afterwards, can be extremely helpful for your relationship with food. To start the process of tuning in, my recommendation is that for the next couple of weeks you ask yourself how hungry you are before you start eating and again halfway through eating, and then how full you are afterwards. This can also be part of the 'mindful eating practice' that I will be talking about next (see page 89).

You can use the scale on the following page to help you frame how you are feeling.

```
├──────────┬──────────┬──────────┬──────────┤
```

Intense hunger   **Hungry**   **Neutral**   **Full**   **Intense fullness**

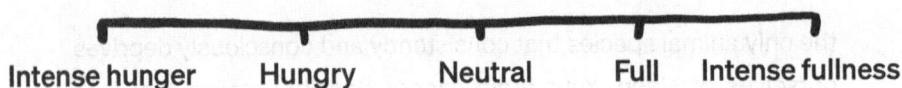

Intense hunger	Irritable, dizzy, nauseous
Hungry	Stomach rumbling, thinking about food, empty stomach
Neutral	Can sense food in stomach, no rumbling
Full	Comfortably full, desire for more food decreased
Intense fullness	Uncomfortable, painful, feel sick, need to unbutton clothing

The key thing to know is that hunger is not your enemy. If you have dieted a lot in the past and followed a lot of prescriptive meal plans, you might have learnt differently — you might have gone through periods of time when you had to ignore your hunger and 'push through' because you weren't 'allowed' to eat yet. When you finally did eat, you would probably have found it really easy to eat more than you needed and beyond the level of feeling satisfied.

My recommendation is to avoid getting too hungry before you eat. When you are feeling hungry and therefore ready to eat, *this* is the time to start thinking about eating. Likewise, when you start to feel like you are getting full, try to stop eating. Know that it can take a while after you finish eating for your 'fullness' signals to kick in, so even after stopping eating you may start to feel even more full.

If you leave it too long before you eat, you may find that you overcompensate by overeating or making food choices that don't feel good to you. If this happens during the day, first up check on the amount of fibre and protein in the meals you had earlier. And think about whether your meals were large enough. Consider adding in a snack if needed. It is better to commit to eating something between meals rather than smashing down a whole packet of crackers and half a block of cheese when you finally get to the fridge and then not enjoying your dinner.

If you find you are hungry at night, start by checking whether you have actually eaten enough during the day. Being hungry in the evening is common if you are 'on a diet' or 'trying to be good', and is something we want to stop happening. It is okay to eat something if you are genuinely hungry and consciously making the decision to eat — this is very different to mindlessly nibbling or picking at food at night when it is cravings that are driving your food choices rather than actual hunger. However, do be aware that if you get into the habit of eating something late every night rather than occasionally, your brain will start to anticipate this happening and can release ghrelin in anticipation — which will then drive you to eat at this time.

Being hungry in the evening and then needing to eat a lot late in the day has happened to me on several occasions when I have been busy and have not eaten enough earlier on. When I consciously shifted things around and ate more in the daytime, I no longer had the desire to eat late and was naturally hungrier during the day.

So, while we need to be in tune with our hunger cues, do also be mindful — they can become dysregulated quite easily based on our daily routines. I will be talking more about this and the timing of eating in Chapter 8.

———————

If you have children, helping them to tune in to their hunger and fullness is a really useful skill to teach them. It can support them to be able to regulate the amount of food they eat in a world where access to food is so easy and regularly eating more than their bodies need can be a real problem.

When it comes to kids, keeping it simple is the best approach. Like others in my profession, I follow the 'division of responsibility' approach of Ellyn Satter (I've listed her website under 'Nutrition' in the resources section on page 295). This invaluable approach follows the principle that you as a caregiver are responsible for *what* and *when* your child eats, and your child is responsible for *how much*. Simple — but incredibly effective. Many of the challenges we as health professionals see these days around children and their eating is a lack of structure and constant grazing without a child truly being able to tune in to their hunger cues.

Since my children were each about four or five, I have asked them before a meal 'How hungry are you, on a scale of 1 to 5?', 5 being super-hungry, and 1 being not so much. This guides me as to how much I initially serve them up (if it is not a 'serve yourself' situation). They are absolutely allowed to leave food on their plates, but they know that if they ask for food an hour later, the same meal (likely cold) will be the only thing on offer. And if there is a lot left on the plate, it will be their lunch the next day heated up and put into one of my food pods for school. No coaxing, no long mealtimes, no negotiations and absolutely never 'eat this and you will get <insert the child's favourite food or dessert here>'. Plain, simple and consistent.

If you have children with sensory needs or highly dysfunctional eating, then a different approach may be required, but for most kids 'back to basics' works. If you need help in this space, my team at Mission Nutrition can help so don't suffer alone here. I know how painful that can be!

Mindful eating

One of the core principles around having a healthy relationship with food is **feeling good about your choices before, during and after you have eaten**. To be able to make that a reality, however, you first need to become more aware of what and how you are eating.

Enter mindful eating. This is the practice of bringing awareness to the thoughts, feelings and sensations that are driving your food choices. And that means really noticing what is going on before, during and after you are eating, which most importantly needs to be done **without judgement**.

It is essential to look at your interactions with food as if you were someone else looking in on the situation. Someone else who is kind, compassionate and supportive, like you would be if you were looking in on your best friend and the way they eat. You wouldn't be mean to them, so you can't be mean to yourself here either!

Having given yourself permission to eat, mindful eating is the next step. It can ultimately support you to make more intentional food choices and to have a greater appreciation of your body and the food you eat, as well as make it easier for you to regulate your desire to eat. By turning inwards and noticing the internal cues and sensations that our bodies give us around the experience of eating, it can be easier to tame binge eating, overeating and eating to manage challenging emotions. So it puts the power back in your hands, rather than you feeling like food has power over you.

But how do you eat mindfully? There are a variety of different ways you can do this, but the following is what I find most helpful.

Initially, practise mindfully eating with a single piece of food when you are on your own with peace and quiet, so you can really engage in the process. Then you can start to integrate the practice into as many meals or snacks as is practical for you in a day, until it eventually becomes second nature for you.

Mindful eating practice

1. **Choose a small piece of food** to do this exercise with. It could be a single raisin, a slice of apple, a spoonful of yoghurt, a

piece of cheese, a cracker or whatever you feel like trying. You can do this exercise repeatedly, so don't overthink your choice about what to eat the first time. Anything will work.

2. Now, close your eyes and turn your attention inwards. Take a few slow, deep breaths to calm your body and mind. **Think about how hungry you are**. Where are the feelings of hunger in your body? What are the physical sensations? Is your stomach feeling empty, rumbling? Now rate your hunger from 1 to 5, with 1 being neutral to very slightly hungry and 5 being intensely hungry.

3. Next, open your eyes. **Look at the food**. Observe the food as if you were looking at it for the first time, with curiosity. Look at its appearance, its shape, its colour. Is it shiny? Steaming? Starting to melt?

4. Now lift it up. **Hold the food**, feel the texture. Is it hard? Is it smooth? Is it rough? Is it firm? Is it soft?

5. Then bring it towards your nose. **What does it smell like?** Is it sweet, salty, earthy, sour, spicy, fragrant? Is the aroma strong or is it faint? If it has no smell at all, just notice that. Notice at the same time if anything is going on in your body. Are you really wanting to take a bite? Are you salivating?

6. Now **place the food in your mouth and notice how it feels**, then chew it slowly and mindfully. Notice the flavour, the texture, and the taste. How would you describe the food? Is it crunchy, smooth, chewy, creamy? Does the flavour tend to change as you continue to chew it and move it around in your mouth? Does it taste different on different parts of your tongue? And as you chew, is there a sound? Is there a crunch? Take as much time as you like.

7. **Swallow the food**, observe what happens to the food, and notice the taste in your mouth afterwards as well as how your body feels.

This is mindful eating in action. Repeat this process with a single food as many times as you like, then start to include this as part of some of your meals until it becomes a habit. It only needs to be the first couple of bites, then noticing how you feel halfway through eating, and then noticing how full you feel afterwards. The aim is to eat until you are satisfied.

To eat mindfully, you don't need to eat on your own or sit in utter silence at every meal! With life as it is, it is unlikely to be practical to do this anyway. It is, however, really helpful to remove distractions while you are eating to at least give you a chance to tune in to your eating. Keep the TV and radio off, your phone off the table, sit down and really commit to the opportunity to enjoy eating. If we eat on the go, eat at our desks and while we are doing other things, it is next to impossible to eat mindfully and truly honour our inbuilt hunger and fullness signals.

Becoming more aware of how you feel before, during and after eating will take time and practice, but when it becomes part of your new normal it can make so much difference. It has completely changed *my* life and my relationship with food! I know it might feel a bit odd at first, but trust the process.

Understanding what's not working for you

There are so many reasons why we eat when we do, many of which have absolutely nothing to do with needing or wanting food. Because we need to eat to live, eating is very habitual, and rightly so. The only challenge is when your habits work *against* you rather than *for* you.

Understanding your patterns of unhelpful eating and identifying the influences on these is the first step when it comes to reprogramming things and getting back to a healthy relationship with food and with your body. I will now take you through some common eating habits and what might drive them.

Autopilot mode

This is the type of eating and drinking many of us do, much of the time. Mindlessly and often unconsciously eating on autopilot and often, this can play into unhelpful eating behaviours.

Here are some different examples of this type of eating.

PICKING AND NIBBLING

This is something I used to have a real issue with. In my teens and twenties, when I was having very small meals and trying to restrict what I was eating, I would frequently end up getting hungry and start picking at things while standing in the kitchen. Somehow this didn't feel the same as committing to a full meal; it kind of didn't count. Although once you added up the ten slivers of cake, a small handful of this and a little nibble of that, I would easily have eaten more than if I'd just allowed myself to commit to a meal in the first place.

In later life, picking and nibbling have shown up when I have needed a break from my screen. It is all too easy to head to the pantry and munch on a few nuts, or a handful of cereal, or those chocolate crispy bites my friend left for the kids, without even noticing, and even if I am not hungry.

Non-hungry eating can happen a lot more when food is in your eye-line or very easy to access, something I learnt the hard way when we moved house. In our old house we used to have all our food in two big cupboards above the kitchen bench. The kitchen was so tiny, there was no room for anything but the kettle to be left out in view. When we moved, however, our kitchen had much larger benches and a couple of open shelves. In an effort to make the new kitchen look nice, I filled them with a variety of jars of different nuts, seeds and dried fruit.

Within a week, I realised that the Brazil nut jar was empty despite us having agreed to only have two a day each because they are so expensive. The cranberries had been demolished, as had the pumpkin seeds. Now, you might be thinking, *nothing wrong with eating some nuts, seeds and a bit of dried fruit, is there?* And the answer is no, nothing too wrong nutrition-wise. The problem was that my husband was just mindlessly eating all these nuts, seeds and dried fruits on top of what he was normally eating during the day, while waiting for the kettle to boil or having a chat on the phone in the kitchen. Looking beyond the expense of those Brazil nuts, he really didn't need that extra food.

The message here is that **there really is a big difference between a handful of nuts, seeds and a bit of dried fruit *mindfully* eaten when you made a conscious decision to put them in your mouth, versus a handful here and a nibble there which don't even register on your radar as having been eaten.**

JUST BECAUSE

It is very easy to eat food or have drinks just because they are 'there', ready for the taking. When you get on a plane, hungry or not, it can be challenging to turn down the seemingly 'free' coffee and cookies on offer. Then there are those 'all you can eat' scenarios with cooked breakfast, cold breakfast and smoothies on offer, all for a fixed price. It feels wrong to not try to get value for money and take most, if not all, of the things, right?

The reality is that there is always a cost to frequently eating extras just because they are 'there', even if the cost isn't monetary. There's nothing fun about feeling uncomfortable, having a sore stomach or your clothes getting tighter over time.

There will always be times when you eat when you don't need to or want to. That's normal and okay; it is when a pattern is happening repeatedly that it becomes unhelpful.

AVOIDING DISCOMFORT

Sometimes we simply can't say 'no thanks' when someone offers us food or drinks. We might feel that we would let someone down, disappoint or offend them by not accepting what they have offered, which can feel uncomfortable.

There are also more difficult scenarios where you have to manage other people who seem to almost intentionally be undermining your efforts to make healthy choices. Your partner bringing home a bag of lollies for you when you had just started a new gym programme and were really keen to break your evening lolly-munching habit. Your workmates insisting that they can't have a glass of wine if you're not having one, too. Or your friend who starts baking and bringing in custard squares the minute you declare you are keen to have more nourishing afternoon tea snacks at work to help you feel and focus better.

Whether deliberately or not, other people can add to your challenges when it comes to eating for the right reasons. There's no use in blaming them, though. **Your job is to make decisions and choices about the way you think and act based on what is right for you, and to have strategies for managing the influence of others.**

It is also important to remember that if someone is offended by you saying 'no thanks' to something when you don't actually need or want it, it is *their* problem to deal with, not yours. Provided that you say no in a nice way, deliver your message confidently and move on swiftly, it should not be an issue. If you have previously always said yes to food/drink or late nights out, it might take a while for people to get used to you changing, but you aren't becoming a different person. You are just developing into a happier, healthier version of yourself.

'What you think about yourself is much more important than what other people think of you.'

— Roman writer Seneca the Elder

AVOIDING WASTE

'Eat up. Think of all those starving children in Africa.' This is something I am sure many of you can relate to. Being forced to clear our plates regardless of whether we needed the food or not, because other people around the world would be grateful to have what we had. I totally get where this narrative came from; it was something I talked to my late grandma about regularly when she was alive. It was so hard living through the war, with ration books and such limited food options — no wonder every meal felt like a gift after that, and wasting food was beyond comprehension.

The challenge, though, is that this deep belief can live on in our lives even when we have food security. Do you still find it hard to leave food on your plate?

We really aren't saving any children around the world by eating more than we need when we aren't hungry — that's done by donating money or resources — so this is a narrative we should change. We need to serve ourselves less, saving excess food for the next day, and allow ourselves to leave the odd thing on our plate even if it is then destined for the compost!

REWARD

'Eat your greens and you can have an ice cream.' 'Finish your homework and I will give you a lollipop.' 'Sit nicely at the optician's and I will buy you a treat.'

I see this in my life every single day as a parent, and honestly it is a nightmare. The use of food as a reward still happens in some schools, as well as in sports, which really makes my blood boil. I know how easy it is to get kids to do what you want when there is a sugary treat at the end of it, and it can become something they soon start to expect all the time.

I am not going to lie; I have got caught in this trap myself. When trying to get my three-year-old son who had broken his arm to sit still so the doctors could put a cast on it, I would have done anything — and a lollipop from the nurses that day was the easiest option. Generally, however, I do everything I can to avoid using food to get my kids to comply.

If this is something you experienced as a child, it may well still be playing out in your life and your eating habits. If you were rewarded or encouraged with food then, now when you have completed a piece of work, done well at something or met a goal, you may well head straight for the bubbles or some celebratory food. Again, sometimes this is fine, but if it becomes a regular occurrence it can turn into a bigger problem.

ASSOCIATIONS

Have you ever seen a child having a meltdown at the supermarket checkout, begging for something from the end of the aisle? Or been to the swimming pool and seen kids drooling over the ice-cream freezer after finishing their lessons, giving the 'Pleeeeeeeeeeease, I will be helpful *all* afternoon' line a go? If you haven't you're in luck, but if you have you will know that these are painful situations to watch and, worse, to experience yourself.

You only have to give in once or twice at the checkout, swimming pool or Mr Whippy van at the beach before children start to associate the activity with the food. And once this is set in place, it then takes being turned down for what seems like at least 50 times before they give up asking. There is nothing wrong with the odd ice cream, of course, but when your child thinks that the van will be delivering the soft white peaks every day of the summer you have a problem on your hands.

These activity–food associations carry through from our childhood to our adult lives, too. Do you always pick up a drink or snack when you get petrol? Buy yourself something tasty for the car ride home after shopping? The sun comes out, and so do the bubbles? If this has become something that happens frequently and feels like you're doing it on autopilot rather than making a conscious choice, it is something to start becoming more aware of.

Regularly eating or drinking things which taste good for five minutes but you really know you didn't need, want or really enjoy, is a habit you can work on reprogramming! More on how to do that is coming soon.

DISTRACTION

It is just so easy to eat mindlessly these days, as there are many distractions. Whether you are eating in front of the TV or while reading emails, the distraction means you aren't aware of what is going into your mouth and how much you are eating. It can be hard for your brain to get you to tune in to its fullness messages when there are lots of other things going on.

That doesn't mean you always have to eat in silence or never eat on the go; it just means that if you can take steps to be more mindful when you are eating, you might find your food choices easier to make.

TRANSITION TIMES

As the end of the day draws near, autopilot mode often gets activated when you are transitioning from one part of the day to another. Whether it has been a difficult day at work, a long day on your own or a chaotic day juggling your kids, it sometimes feels like the pantry door opens on its own and the chippies/crackers/tasty salty snacks just hop into your mouth without you feeling like you even made the decision to open the packets! The end of the day can also be the time when wine seems to make its way into glasses without you noticing that you're pouring it.

As the day goes on, you become more tired, your willpower declines, and your decisions around what you eat and drink can easily become less and less intentional.

Reactive response

Alongside the many types of 'autopilot mode' eating and drinking, there is what I like to call 'reactive response'. This means eating or drinking as a direct result of trying to manage an emotional state that you are finding challenging at the time.

The terms 'emotional eating' or 'comfort eating' are often used for this, but to me these phrases feel so deeply linked with the vision of a girl breaking up with her boyfriend and digging into a litre container of ice cream that they're not very helpful. *Bridget Jones's Diary* might have played a part here.

Eating or drinking in response to a challenging emotional state is so much more than dealing with just one of the emotions — like sadness — and trying to drown your sorrows or cheer yourself up.

You can also react this way when you experience emotions like loneliness, anger, frustration, overwhelm, anxiety or fatigue. And often this type of eating and drinking doesn't make you feel better or give you comfort at all. More often, the whole situation makes you feel much worse; it can sometimes be more like a form of self-punishment than self-support.

It is normal to have some degree of reactive response eating/drinking — and again, it is only when this becomes a strong pattern and starts affecting your life and your relationships that it becomes a signal that changes need to happen.

Many of the eating challenges I shared in my story at the beginning of the book were anchored in this reactive response. After endless years of dieting and restriction, I turned to food and alcohol to cope whenever challenging emotions raised their heads. At university I remember this all too well. After my school playground days, rejection had become a huge trigger for me. If there was ever a sniff of conflict between my friends or I had a heated discussion with my boyfriend at the time over just about anything, I would be straight into the kitchen, eating dry cereal out of the box, slicing pieces of cheese that I didn't even like, and tearing off tiny pieces of malt loaf until after 15 minutes I had eaten it all and opened another packet.

Alcohol is something I used to struggle with, too. It was the first port of call when I was feeling stressed or overwhelmed about pretty much anything! This was a pattern that became far too frequent and one which I carried a lot of shame about at the time.

If you, too, are doing things like this, please know you are not bad, stupid or ridiculous. You have simply subconsciously learnt to use food and drink for something it was not designed to be used for. Just like I did.

The good news is that now you know this, like me you can change it. So, let's find some solutions for you.

Chapter 5
Reprogramming unhelpful habits

When it comes to reprogramming the unhelpful behaviours you have that mean you are eating when you aren't hungry, or having more than you wanted, or are sabotaging your wellbeing with the way you are drinking, first up you need to remember this: **you are a HUMAN BEING, not a robot, and you need to treat yourself accordingly**. It isn't possible to simply pop in a microchip that will ensure you say 'no thanks' to cake when you don't really want it, skip the crackers when you are feeling bored, or pass on that third glass of wine when you are stressed.

It also isn't possible to change everything at once, so try to work on one thing at a time.

This reprogramming requires you to invest in yourself, do the work to get to the bottom of what is driving your unhelpful eating, and then rewire it by practising new, more helpful behaviours over and over again until they become second nature. And it doesn't only work for behaviours you have around food. This is the very reprogramming process I have followed to break my own cycles of self-destruction. It has helped me stop bingeing, manage my anxiety, reduce my drinking, deal with stress, scroll less often on my phone, and redirect my reactions in pressured situations.

Here is how it is done: four steps of **awareness**, **reflection**, **labelling** the habit and then **creating a plan**!

I have used this four-step process time and time again to help people reprogram their unhelpful behaviours. It is based on the principles of the habit loop that we talked about on page 37. There is a downloadable template on my website that takes you through all four steps: www.claireturnbull.co.nz/endyourfightwithfood.

Step 1: Awareness

Awareness is the first stage of change. You need to become fully aware of your unhelpful eating or drinking behaviours and what is dragging you into them. This is a practice that takes time but is an absolute game-changer.

One of the best ways to become aware of what you are doing is by writing it down. Putting pen to paper. The process of physically writing things down — rather than typing them out or just thinking about them when you are driving — means you become fully committed to the process. When you can see things in black and white on a page, it allows you to separate yourself from them and gives you the opportunity to enter the next step of the process, which is reflection.

ACTION TIME! Keep a diary for at least seven days, ideally longer, of everything you eat and drink. Either as you add in the details or at the end of the day, go back through the diary and identify whether you were eating based on response to genuine hunger, or if there was an aspect of some autopilot mode being activated and/or a reactive response. Consider the same sort of thing for drinking, too.

Then add a few more that capture what was going on at the time. Why do you think you ate or drank what you did? How were you feeling? What were you thinking? Your notes will likely be different for each situation — that's fine, just note down what feels relevant to you.

Finally, note the occasions where the eating/drinking was in some part an unhelpful habit — for example, you ate far more than you wanted to, or you weren't hungry, or you were trying to manage your feelings. If restriction was part of this, note that down, too. Finally, also note whether this was an unhelpful pattern that repeated itself.

To make this easier, you can download a template for your awareness diary from my website. On the opposite page is an example of how some diary entries might look.

The goal here is to identify the behaviours which are problematic for *you*. Please don't judge the nutritional value of what you are eating or think you need to start counting calories — that is not what this process is about. The reason we are looking at this now, before the chapter which covers 'what to eat', is that we need to discover our eating patterns so we can reprogram them *first*. If you do this, then if these old habits crop up when you start making adjustments to improve your nutrition, you will have the tools and skills you need to manage them.

Monday 24th				
Time	6 a.m.	8.30 a.m.	10.20 a.m.	...
What I ate/drank	Tea, muesli/ yoghurt/ berries.	Latte and 4 marshmallows.	Glass of water and 3 cookies.	...
Location	Kitchen.	Coffee shop.	Office kitchen.	...
What type of eating was this?*	Genuine hunger.	Genuine hunger + autopilot.	Reactive response.	...
Why did I eat this?	My normal morning routine.	I wanted the coffee, but just had the marshmallows because they were there and they were free. I ate them while I was waiting.	Got a really rude email from a customer and was feeling angry about it. Needed a break, so went to the kitchen for a glass of water but then saw the cookies.	...
What was I thinking and feeling at the time?	Was just thinking about getting out the door.	First marshmallow was okay, didn't enjoy the others. Thinking about everything I had to do, very distracted. In honesty, I don't even remember consciously picking them up.	Angry and wanting something sweet to eat.	...
Unhelpful pattern?	No, all good.	Yes. Mindless eating.	Yes. When I'm angry, I often eat sweet food.	...

* For this choose between 'genuine hunger', 'autopilot' and 'reactive response'.

KEY MESSAGE

Remember that awareness is the first stage of change, and without it nothing can happen.

As you go through this process, as with the mindful eating exercise on page 89, it is essential for you to apply **self-compassion**. This is not a process of judgement, and the more honest you can allow yourself to be, then the easier it will be to fix things.

It is also helpful to know that keeping a record of your behaviour to increase your awareness of it is something you can return to at any time. I still do this now, from time to time, if I notice unhelpful eating behaviours creeping back in or I have challenges with any of my other behaviours (be that being overly reactive to my kids and husband, or spending too much time on my phone). This approach works for all sorts of behaviours. Life happens and things change, so there will always be times when you need to revisit this — keep it in your tool kit.

Step 2: Reflection

The second step in the reprogramming process is to reflect on the notes you made in your awareness diary. Highlight or circle the patterns that showed up repeatedly in the seven or so days you did your diary for. You will likely notice some eating patterns that are habitual and no problem at all, like having breakfast before work or making a snack when you are genuinely hungry. You might also see patterns where you are eating or drinking for genuine enjoyment. Again, those aren't unhelpful eating behaviours.

If you pick up any restrictive eating situations, like only having a small meal at dinnertime because you ate cookies earlier in the day, head back to pages 81–82 and use this as an opportunity to work through the questions I asked there. **The patterns we are looking at reprogramming here are the mindless autopilot eating/drinking or reactive response type which aren't working for you.**

Once you have identified the eating/drinking patterns you want to reprogram, the next step is to break down each into its habit loop to see what is sitting underneath and driving the behaviour.

Here is a recap on what a habit loop looks like:

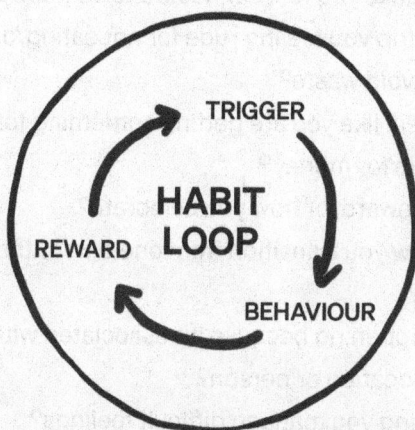

The trigger

Firstly, think about the trigger or triggers for each eating pattern you want to change. Where is this happening? Is it always at work? Always in your kitchen? In the mornings? When you drive a certain way home? When a certain person talks to you? When you do school pick-up? When you're feeling overwhelmed? Tired? Frustrated?

The reward

Next, work out what you are getting out of each unhelpful eating pattern. It might be one thing every time; it might be several. Every default pattern has at least a couple of layers and will serve a purpose; the trick is working out what that is.

Ask yourself: What is the benefit of this pattern? As part of this, you might want to think about how it's related to the different types of autopilot eating and the reactive response eating outlined in Chapter 4 (see pages 92–99).

- Is it something you do to pass the time? A distraction?
- Is it happening without you realising? Mindlessness?
- Does it make you feel connected to someone else?
- Does it stop you feeling rude for not eating/drinking?
- Does it avoid waste?
- Does it feel like you are getting something for free? Or the best value for money?
- Is this a reward, or how you celebrate?
- Is this how you transition from one part of the day to another?
- Is this happening because it's associated with a particular activity, location or person?
- Is it helping you manage difficult feelings?
- Does it confirm a belief you have — for example, having no willpower?
- Is it a form of self-sabotage?

Sometimes the reward is very straightforward; other times it is a little more complex. Especially if you are doing something that makes you feel worse afterwards. Could it be that you're doing this because it confirms what you believe to be true about yourself?

That you have no self-control? That you aren't good enough? That no one cares? **Be kind to yourself here. This can be tough stuff to look at.**

As you work through your patterns, really dig deep and look at what is underneath — because until you find the things that are driving you to do what you do, you will be forever at the mercy of your habit loops driving you in an unhelpful direction.

My own experience: One of the patterns I had in my late thirties was having alcohol every night of the week; something I never did in my twenties or early thirties. When I identified this as a habit I wanted to change, I filled in this awareness diary for a few weeks so I could start looking at what was going on in the habit loop.

The trigger was easy: shutting down my laptop. It was like closing the lid signified that my work phase was over for at least the next hour while I moved on to doing things with the kids. It took me a long time to get to the root of the *reward* I was getting from the behaviour, but when I finally got there I realised it was multi-layered.

Firstly, as I work from home a lot of the time, it was acting as a signal that I was transitioning from one part of my life to another in the same space. Secondly, I never drink when I am working, so having a drink was giving me permission to 'clock off', at least for a while. I admit that at different stages of my life I have been addicted to work, as was my dad who I saw model this as normal behaviour; so doing something that allowed me to disconnect from that work addiction was powerful and ended up being addictive in its own way!

Thirdly, having that drink was something for me alone — it required no one's input, no one's opinion, and didn't require me to have to think about the needs of others, which I constantly do all the time in every other aspect of my life. Like so many working mums, in adjusting to the juggle of working *and* looking after kids, I lost myself; and for a while I found that alcohol was like a Band-Aid to deal with the stress.

So, there were a lot of rewards; and when I was able to look at my habit loop like this, I was able to see why it was so hard for me to stop. It also showed me that I needed to find other ways to deal with the challenges I was facing without having a drink. I rewired this habit using the rest of the steps in the process, and now it is something that I manage well most of the time.

Step 3: Label it

Once you have been through the habit loop for each unhelpful behaviour and worked out what the triggers and rewards are, there comes another, very important step. Name the patterns or label each of them in some way that is meaningful to you. You might find pictures, a key ring or changing the wallpaper on your phone to an image of what you are using as your label helpful to act as a reminder.

This was something I did in my earlier years to reprogram my habit of bingeing. It was suggested to me by a health professional called Debbie who I was working with. She suggested that I create a character for my unhelpful habit. So I drew a picture, the picture opposite in fact. It was a grumpy and sad-looking guy who I felt represented how I was feeling any time I was about to binge. Debbie suggested I give him a name and I came up with Percy.

I kept this picture visible in my bedroom, where my bingeing habit would most often start off — negative thoughts when I was sitting on my own that drove me to the kitchen cupboards. The picture reminded me that when my habit loop was getting triggered, it was simply that 'Percy' was being activated and I wasn't to blame.

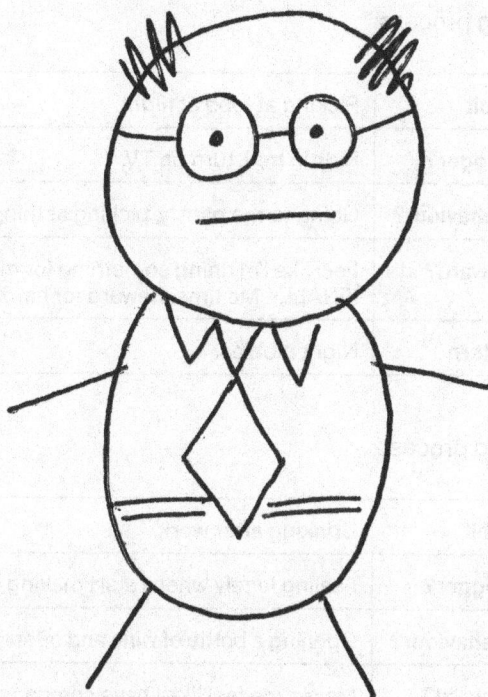

Doing this labelling helps separate *you* from *your behaviour* and it is one of the most helpful tools I have ever learnt to use, especially because self-blame and shame only fuel the cycle of unhelpful behaviours. While we are responsible for reworking our unhelpful habits, if we think that *we* are the problem, rather than *the behaviour* being the problem, this does nothing to help break the cycle.

Please, however, avoid naming or labelling your patterns after anyone you know or someone you dislike — that activates blame, which is not the intention here.

On the following page are a couple of examples of how labelling works.

Fran's labelling process:

Repeating habit	Picking at food at night.
What is the trigger?	Kids in bed, turn on TV.
What is the behaviour?	Going to the pantry, picking at things.
What is the reward?	Feel like I'm doing something for myself FINALLY. Me time. Reward for hard day.
Name the pattern	Night nibbles.

Sam's labelling process:

Repeating habit	Drinking after work.
What is the trigger?	Feeling lonely when I start making dinner.
What is the behaviour?	Opening a bottle of wine and often finishing it.
What is the reward?	Makes me feel like I have company. Makes me forget what I'm worried about.
Name the pattern	Lonely drinking.

Step 4: Create a plan

Once you have collected all of the details about your habit loops and labelled them, it's time to start changing them with an action plan. There are three parts to this step:

1. Firstly, do whatever you possibly can to reduce the likelihood of the trigger being activated. The more you do this, the easier it will be to avoid being dragged around the loop.
2. Secondly, make the behaviour harder to do.

3. Thirdly, figure out what you will do instead of the behaviour you are looking to avoid, if and when you are triggered. It is highly likely that this will happen sometimes, so it is best to be prepared! You also want to make sure you make the alternative behaviour as easy as possible to happen.

When it comes to this part, you can do the work to figure out a plan for each of the unhelpful habits you have identified, but then it's best to put one plan into action at a time. When you have nailed that one, move on to the next. It is often best to start with the easiest one first so that you feel like you are winning!

I've given examples below from two people struggling with different things, and then I've gone into more detail about how to achieve each part of this step.

Fran's plan:

Name of pattern	Night nibbles.
Reducing trigger activation	Watch TV in another room so I don't walk through the kitchen.
Making the behaviour harder	Put the foods I nibble on higher up or out of reach.
What I could do instead, to feel how I really want to feel	This is really about me wanting my own time, space, and something for myself. Write a list of things I can do that make me feel like me, and do one of those a night, e.g. paint nails, do Sudoku.
Notes	I also need to talk to my husband about not bringing snacks to me during the evening because I find it hard to say no when the chips are already in the bowl!

Sam's plan:

Name of pattern	Lonely drinking.
Reducing trigger activation	Stop buying wine when I go to the supermarket each week.
Making the behaviour harder	Watch a cooking programme while I am making dinner.
What I could do instead, to feel how I really want to feel	Arrange calls with my friends during the week, to look forward to. Get back into netball and rejoin the team I used to be part of.
Notes	I never used to feel lonely. I think I have lost confidence to reach out to people. I really want to change this pattern.

1. Reduce trigger activation

As I said earlier, habit triggers can be environmental cues such as specific locations, times of day, objects, people or emotional states. They can also be a combination of these — like, you are in your kitchen (location), in the morning (time: 6–7 a.m.), feeling overwhelmed about the day ahead (emotional state), and you have that third coffee despite knowing it's not helpful or what you want to be doing.

LOCATION, TIME, OBJECT AND PEOPLE TRIGGERS
Examples of trigger activations around food might be:

- Entering your kitchen, making you feel like you need to eat or drink something.
- Going to your local pub and feeling the social pressure to drink.
- Children going to bed, finally getting time to yourself, so the

desire to eat or drink kicks in.
- Seeing biscuits in the pantry and feeling the desire to eat them.
- Passing your local cafe and heading in to check out the latest bakery items.
- Catching up with your friend and over-ordering food, as you always do together.
- Attending a work function and avoiding awkward conversations by drinking or eating.

Here are some examples of things that trigger other unhelpful behaviours:

- Standing in a room that triggers feelings of anxiety or stress due to past negative experiences.
- Getting into bed and picking up your phone.
- Going to your in-laws' place and eating excessively to be polite.
- Your phone vibrating, so you pick it up to check what is happening.

TIME TO REFLECT: Have a think about what triggers your unhelpful behaviours. Is there anything you can do to reduce how often you experience these triggers? Or how you could manage these triggers?

EMOTIONAL STATE TRIGGERS
The emotions you experience can have a huge influence on your eating and drinking behaviour. When you experience a particular emotional state over and over again, it is easy to create a 'habit loop' to help manage that emotion, and this can sometimes play out in the form of unhelpful behaviour.

If, however, you can name the emotional state you're experiencing, this can help you tame it and find a way to work through the process of managing it *without* turning to food or drink. Much like the labelling of a habit (like my friend Percy), naming your emotional state at the time helps you separate *you* from *the emotions* so you can be more objective about the situation.

ACTION TIME! Reflecting on the unhelpful eating behaviours you have identified so far, what emotions do you think crop up when they are happening? Look at the emotions listed below and see if some words jump out at you. More often than not, problem eating is associated with negative emotions, so I have given more examples of those than positive ones. There may be other words in your mix, too — if they resonate better, choose those.

angry	pessimistic	excited
apathetic	sad	cheerful
frustrated	bored	optimistic
stressed	lonely	joyful
nervous	disheartened	grateful
worried	tired	happy
anxious	depressed	proud
irritated	exhausted	at ease
disappointed	drained	calm

MANAGING EMOTIONAL STATES

Once you have identified the emotions that are associated with your unhelpful habits, you are all set to create a plan for managing them in the moment without the need to turn to food or drink.

Here are some ideas to try!

* Move your body: We can learn a lot from animals when it comes to the value of moving your body to process difficulties. Have you ever seen ducks after they have had a fight? They often furiously flap their wings, which is believed to let them release stress from their bodies after the confrontation; and then they get on with life like nothing had ever happened.

Clearly our brains are very different to the ones ducks have, but there is still a lesson here. The ducks move their bodies while processing what they have experienced; their movement diffuses the energy and then they move on to the next thing.

Rather than turning to food or drink when you experience strong or challenging emotions, finding a way to move your body can really help you work through the peak of the emotions when they feel like they are taking you over.

For me, movement has been an essential part of managing my emotional states and overcoming my eating issues. In my late twenties I started to notice the agitation in my body when I was feeling stressed, anxious and apprehensive. I learnt to get my trainers on and go for a quick run around the block, and it worked every time. I hit a stumbling block when I had kids, though, as I couldn't just leave the house if the kids were eating or sleeping or I was waiting for someone to arrive. So I had to find another solution, which was doing ten press-ups, ten star-jumps and ten squats whenever I felt any overwhelming emotions come up. Or running up and down the corridor 20 times. It does take practice for movement to become a new habit, but I promise you it works!

If your emotion is a positive one, like you are excited, and you tend to celebrate with eating, again movement can help. A good dance to help process that excitement might be just what you need to get into a better space. It's easier to make helpful eating and drinking choices after your emotion has peaked and calmed.

I will talk more about the benefits of movement in Chapter 9.

ACTION TIME! What kind of movement would work for you in your situation? It is important to be as specific as possible here rather than just telling yourself you will move when you feel stressed — that will likely not happen.

- Could you walk or run up and down the stairs at work, or go around the block, if you feel yourself experiencing overwhelm and heading for the biscuit tin?
- Could you put a sign somewhere in your kitchen that says 'jog on the spot' so that you get that done before you decide whether you actually need to start eating because you are bored?
- Could you put weights by your desk and do 30 bicep curls and 30 squats when you feel like heading upstairs for that fifth coffee you don't really need or you're picking up your phone for the hundredth time that day?

∗**Listen to music:** Music has a powerful ability to change your emotional state, and as such it can be an extremely useful tool. It is also so accessible these days; you can play it almost any time, wherever you are, if you have your phone and a pair of headphones. If I am feeling exhausted, which is a trigger for me to eat something to try to perk myself up, the right music can help me manage this feeling and reduce my need to raid the fridge.

If you are feeling stressed and overwhelmed, calmer music with a slower tempo can really help. When my kids are running around the house (even after plenty of time on the trampoline or wrestling, as boys do), I often put on hip hop lofi beats, a chilled music album or acoustic tunes to calm the mood; and for the most part, it is quite effective.

If you are feeling a bit flat, sad or bored, some more upbeat, higher-tempo music might be just the ticket to help you feel better. To enhance the effectiveness, if you can get up and move around to the music, then you will get the added benefit of movement along with the good vibes from the tunes.

If music doesn't do it for you, then listening to or watching something funny might work. It is all about finding the right solution for *you*!

ACTION TIME! Set up some playlists to put on when you notice the emotions arising that are associated with your unhelpful habits. You can use the same names as you gave your habit loops as an easy reminder. For the bingeing habit loop I had, 'Claire's Percy playlist' would have been a good name.

★ Breathing: The quickest and easiest way to take control of your emotions is to control your breathing. When you are experiencing strong emotions, you may find your breaths becoming shorter and shallower, which is communicating to your brain that you are in danger. This, in turn, may heighten the strength of the emotion and make things worse, possibly driving you even more compellingly towards unhelpful behaviour.

In contrast, doing some slow, intentional diaphragmatic breathing can calm your nervous system and put you more in tune with your body so you are able to create the space to be more intentional about your behaviour. Essentially, this can increase the gap between the trigger and the behaviour by allowing you to be more mindful about what is going on.

ACTION TIME! There are all sorts of different breathing practices you can try when you are working through strong emotions — see page 242 where I go through one of these in detail.

✱**Progressive muscle relaxation:** When strong emotions take hold, it can make you feel very disconnected from your body. One tool I have found very helpful is called progressive muscle relaxation, a technique developed by Dr Edmund Jacobson in the early twentieth century. It involves systematically tensing and then relaxing different muscle groups in the body, typically starting with the feet. You tense the muscles in your feet for 5–10 seconds before relaxing them completely. You then move up through your body, repeating the same process with your calves, thighs, abdomen, arms, hands, shoulders and face. This can be an effective way to alleviate feelings associated with stress and bring about calm in your body.

ACTION TIME! Have a go at doing this technique and see how you feel afterwards. Could it be something you could use to help you manage some of your unhelpful habit loops?

✱**Get outside:** Even five minutes spent standing outside in the fresh air with natural light getting into your eyes can significantly change how you feel. If it is longer, or you are moving at the same time, it is even better. Connecting your bare feet with the ground outside has also been shown to be helpful for some people. If you are able to take your shoes off and stand on the grass, on rock or even on sand, if that is accessible to you, it can be a game-changer!

If strong emotions take hold, this is a fantastic tool to have in your kit to break the cycle and move away from any unhelpful behaviours you are trying to rewire.

ACTION TIME! Think about your unhelpful habits. Could getting outside when challenging emotions arise be a strategy you could apply for any of the patterns you are working on? Could it become a new, helpful habit?

* **Shift your focus:** What you experience internally includes your thoughts, emotions and physical sensations. Your *external* experience, on the other hand, includes anything you can sense via your five senses — so what you can see, hear, taste, smell and touch. If you are able to shift your experience from internal to external this can help you become more aware of what is going on and enable you to then take control of your behaviour.

ACTION TIME! Where you are right now, stop and think about what you can see. What can you hear? What can you taste? Smell? Touch? Become aware of what is going on around you.

Set a time in your calendar to practise this every day for a week, and see if it is something you feel could work as a tool to help you manage your triggers for the unhelpful habits you are looking to reprogram.

* **Get it out of your head:** Writing down your thoughts and feelings or talking them through with someone else can be extremely helpful; it is something I cannot recommend highly enough. Processing things in this way — rather than letting the thoughts go round and round in your head — can help reduce feelings of anxiety and overwhelm. It also encourages awareness, which helps you the *next* time these challenging emotions come up. You will find it easier to see a pattern emerging if you have previously captured it, especially if you have written it down and can see the words in your own handwriting.

ACTION TIME! Do this now, so you're ready when a strong emotion hits and spins you around:

1. Get a journal or pad of paper and a pen, and place it in the location where your unhelpful habit unfolds. If this is in the kitchen, put it there. If things start off in your office, put it there. Make sure it is obvious and accessible.
2. Think of one or two people you could contact if strong emotions, thoughts or triggers arise, then contact them and let them know your plan and line them up to help. If they aren't there at the time you call, no worries — default to writing your thoughts and feelings down to get the stuff out of your head!

WHEN TO SEEK ADDITIONAL HELP

While it is very normal to experience a range of emotions each day, things can get out of balance, and it may be best to seek professional support. I have done so several times in my life.

This could be the case if you are feeling strong emotions that persist — for example, an ongoing sense of hopelessness or despair. Or feelings that interfere with your ability to live your life — for example, feeling so anxious that you are almost unable to leave the house. Or feelings that are out of proportion to what most people would feel in that situation — for example, always feeling 'on guard' or fearful.

Please seek personalised help from a qualified health professional such as your GP rather than try to push through. There is also a list of helpline numbers in the resources section on page 297.

2. Make the behaviour harder to do and less appealing

When you're 'in' a habit loop, it can feel like there is no time between you experiencing your trigger and the behaviour happening. Often it is not until you sit down with the glass of wine in your hand that you realise that, somehow, on autopilot, you must have walked through the door, put your bag down and poured out a glass like you were in some kind of time warp.

To reduce the likelihood of this automatic reaction happening, it is extremely helpful to put barriers in place that make it harder for you to do the behaviour automatically. Essentially, this is putting a gap between the trigger and the behaviour — what I like to call the *magic second*. This is the second when your action can go from being a subconscious one to a conscious one.

Over time, this second can grow from one to two and beyond, giving you more time to make a conscious decision about what to do.

The first time I realised the power of this technique was when we moved house nine years ago. In our old house we had a battered

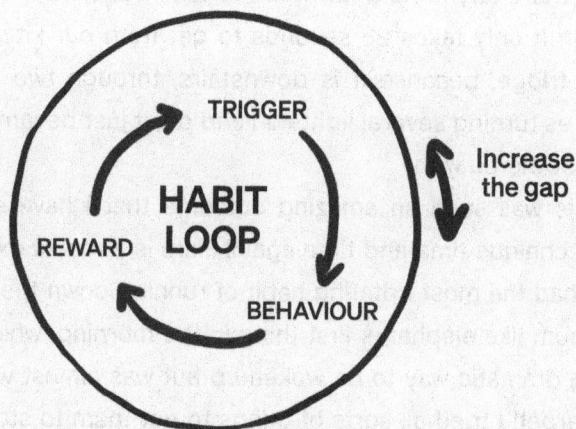

121

old fridge under cover outside the back door which held extra milk and cold drinks, including beer. Despite the front door being the obvious access to the house, when my husband got home from work he always walked through the garden to check how things were looking and came in through the back door. After a while, I noticed him starting to come in through the back door with a bottle of beer in his hand, which he had picked up on his way past the fridge — in this case, his trigger.

One beer down, he would often get another while he was working on wrapping up his emails and dinner prep was under way. Sometimes, if the day had been a stressful one, a third one was opened. A strong habit loop had been unintentionally created. He would often say to me that he didn't even really want it, but that wasn't until he was halfway through a bottle.

I didn't think much of it at the time, but when we moved house the battered old fridge ended up in the garage downstairs, with our kitchen and living area upstairs. For the first couple of weeks, my husband did sometimes head downstairs to get a beer, but the days gradually got further apart, until — quite unintentionally — he just stopped drinking midweek because the trigger wasn't really there anymore, and the behaviour was harder to do. Even though it only takes 23 seconds to get from our kitchen to the other fridge, because it is downstairs, through two doors and requires turning several lights on and off, it just became too hard to be bothered with.

This was such an amazing outcome that I have since used this technique time and time again! Here is a recent example. My boys had the most irritating habit of running down the hallway to our room like elephants first thing in the morning, which was not only a dramatic way to be woken up but was almost wearing out the carpet! I tried all sorts of things to get them to stop doing it. Asking them nicely, for several months, was the first step, but as you probably can imagine, that really wasn't that effective. The next step was to make it lighter in the corridor, as they said one of the reasons they did it was to get to us as fast as possible because it was dark. That kind of worked for a while. But by this point, light on or not, the running was a habit that had become so entrenched that stronger action needed to be taken.

So, I put a large basket in the middle of the corridor. This *forced* them to not run down the corridor. Seeing the basket increased the gap between the trigger (coming out of their bedroom in the morning) and the behaviour (running). After about two weeks they stopped running down the corridor. After that I intermittently put it back, as old habits can easily creep back in; but now, over 18 months later, things are 99% better — all because I made it HARDER for them to do what they were doing.

3. Alternative response: a new habit instead

Hopefully, if you put parts 1 and 2 above into action, you will be less likely be triggered and therefore will not put your unhelpful behaviour into action. However, you still need a plan for when you *do* get triggered as this will no doubt happen from time to time.

Using an alternative response is like carving out a new pathway. Initially it might be hard to create the path, especially if there is long grass and lots of weeds, but over time, when you tread that path repeatedly, it becomes more obvious and easier to walk through.

This is the approach I implemented as a way to stall my binges. Over time, I had become more aware of the triggers for my binges — being in the house on my own, feeling lonely and like I didn't know what to do with myself — which would normally then lead to me heading to the dairy to get some family-sized bags of chocolates, or going downstairs and picking at food, or baking and eating most of the mixture before it got cooked.

I decided I would start having a shower to begin breaking this cycle. Initially it was mid-binge; then, as I became more aware of my behaviours, it was after I had bought the chocolate but before I had eaten it. Then I was able to shower before I went to the shops or downstairs; and finally, after a few years, I was able to do it as soon as I started to become aware of the triggers kicking in.

It was so effective. It broke the cycle, and allowed the waves of emotion to peak and then fall away.

With all alternative responses, you also need to make them as easy to do as possible. I talk about this when I look at building helpful habits in Chapter 9 (see page 213).

Putting it all together

On the opposite page there are a couple of examples of working through the four-step process to reprogram unhelpful behaviour.

Bonus tip: Be aware of *why* you might have got into a particular habit. It might be because you want to make sure you get your fair share; maybe as a child you always got less than your siblings. It could also be that you don't want anything to be wasted.

Moana's four-step process:

1	Unhelpful habit (awareness)	Always feeling like I need to finish all the food I cooked for dinner. Eating all the leftovers while I tidy up. Feel uncomfortably full and bloated afterwards and annoyed at myself.
2	Triggers (reflection)	Seeing food left on the bench after everyone has finished eating.
3	Label	The leftover trap.
4 (Plan)	1. Reduce trigger activations	When I am serving up the meals for everyone, put any leftovers on a separate plate and cover it so it is less tempting to eat when I have already had my dinner and I am full.
	2. Make it harder	Put the leftovers in the fridge before I start washing up so I don't see them.
	3. New habit instead	Have the leftovers for lunch the next day.

Robin's four-step process:

1	Unhelpful habit (awareness)	Stopping by the petrol station on the way home and picking up something to eat in the car even though I don't really need or want it. Also spending money I don't want to on this daily habit.
2	Triggers (reflection)	Driving past the petrol station on my way home.
3	Label	Snack-stop.
4 (Plan)	1. Reduce trigger activations	Drive a different way home.
	2. Make it harder	When I do need to go there to buy petrol, use the pay-at-the-pump service and avoid going into the store.
	3. New habit instead	Take a snack to work to eat in the car on the way home if I am hungry and need to eat something.

'I decry the injustice of my wounds, only to look down and see that I am holding a smoking gun in one hand and a fistful of ammunition in the other.'

— professional counsellor
Craig D. Lounsbrough

Addressing self-sabotage

One thing to work through on your journey to improve your relationship with food and with yourself is **addressing any aspects of self-sabotage**. This was one of the things that used to bother me the most when it came to my own eating issues. Why was it that sometimes I almost deliberately ate more than I needed, or consciously bought that extra bag of Maltesers when I already had two in my hand? There were definitely times when I felt so bad about myself that I intentionally went out to buy lots of chocolate — knowing full well it would make me feel worse, not better, after eating it. Self-sabotage in action.

This is something we often do outside of the realm of food, too. It is common to sabotage relationships, work opportunities and things we enjoy even when they are going well. That feels like it doesn't make sense, right? Why do we sometimes almost intentionally make things more difficult for ourselves?

However, it does make sense when you look at the psychology behind it. Self-sabotage is psychological self-harm — it feels safe to experience something familiar, even if that something is painful and uncomfortable. Also, we experience what is known as confirmation bias — we seek to find things we believe to be true rather than seeking for evidence to support a new story. If, say, you believe you are undeserving of love, then you will subconsciously make sure you don't get it by pushing people away.

I have several good friends who were brought up in abusive family environments and have then ended up in abusive relationships themselves, because it feels familiar and, in some screwed-up way, on some level it feels 'safe' to them. When you're a child, it is safer to believe that *you* are the problem rather than your caregivers, because (unlike many other animals) young humans rely on older humans to survive. Children who are being abused often aren't able to see that it is their caregivers who are at fault; it is safer for these children to believe that they are the ones who are to blame for being hit, verbally attacked or hurt in some other way. As adults, they then accept and excuse the behaviour of the other people in their lives who abuse them, because it is a story they are used to. A tragic case of 'better the devil you know'.

Sometimes, too, we self-sabotage when we lack self-confidence. I have worked with clients who have sabotaged job opportunities by turning up late to interviews or not doing the prep for an exam even though they really want to pass, because in some way this confirms their belief that they aren't good enough for the job or smart enough to pass the exam. This could be because of things they were told by other people earlier in their lives, or because of self-imposed pressure and expectations to be perfect. Many of these same clients were also deliberately eating and drinking more than they wanted or needed to because this was another action that supported the narrative that they weren't good enough to take care of their body.

If you sabotage things in your life, please know you are not alone. You are normal — it is part of being human to have created patterns that your brain believes serve you.

———

To get away from self-sabotage, you need to first become aware that it's happening, and that it is just another unhelpful habit to reprogram. Look to find the triggers and the patterns. Journalling, mindfulness or therapy can all help you uncover the underlying beliefs or fears that are driving your self-sabotaging behaviour.

Next comes challenging those negative thoughts and beliefs, which I will talk about in Chapter 11 (see page 259). By questioning and reframing negative self-talk, along with creating new affirmations and beliefs, you can work to resolve self-sabotage. Also, practising self-care and stress management techniques, which we will come to soon, will help. Prioritising rest, relaxation and activities that bring you joy and fulfilment supports your overall wellbeing and resilience in the face of setbacks.

You deserve love, joy, peace and support in your life, and you are good enough just the way you are. My goal is to get you to believe that because I know it is true.

'We sabotage the great things in our lives because deep down, we don't feel worth having the great things.'

— life coach Taressa Riazzi

If you have had issues with doing things on autopilot, or as a reactive response, or self-sabotage or other similar challenges for years (or indeed much of your life), you need to accept that **the process of reprogramming yourself will take time**. You are a human being, after all, not a robot.

If you learnt to drive on the left-hand side of the road and travel to another country where they also drive on the left, the transition will be easy for you. Apart from the odd difference in road rules, you approach roundabouts in the same way, get off highways in the same way and overtake in the same way. Your default programming makes driving something that happens without much, if any, conscious thought. If, however, you go to a country where they drive on the other side of the road, it will take months, if not years, for this to become completely normal for you. Initially, it will take a lot of concentration and conscious thought to make it happen.

My brother experienced this phenomenon when he moved to France and had to drive on the other side of the road. On several occasions he had some near-misses when his brain was in autopilot mode. He ended up putting a big Post-It note on his dashboard with an arrow drawn on it to visually remind him to stay on the right-hand side! Now, years later, it is completely normal for him to drive on the right — so much so that when he was last in the UK with me, we pulled out of a car park and went to move to the right side of the road, and I had to shout very loudly to remind him to stay on the left!

Be it reprogramming unhelpful habits or building yourself new helpful ones, which we will be coming to soon (see page 207), the key message is that it takes time. That is why 6-week crash diets or 12-week programmes so often fail — there just isn't enough time for you to embed new habits into your life. So cut yourself some slack, change your mental approach to this process, and see it as a journey of self-discovery and opportunity rather than a focused few weeks that will fix things. It won't. Going for a 'quick fix' will only lead to disappointment and make you feel like you have failed.

I like to think of the journey of change as being a bit like a series of waves — it certainly was for me. Initially the waves were big, and really up and down sometimes. I would have things sussed for a few weeks, then I would binge and binge again, then work myself back to a better space. Over time, though, the binges got smaller and less frequent — the waves began to calm. I was able to accept that the up-and-down waves are all part of the process and that a couple of binges didn't mean anything, that it was just an opportunity to learn more about myself and more about my triggers. This acceptance meant it was easier to get back into a routine and move on with my new healthy habits. The ups and downs are an essential part of the reprogramming process.

Even when the waves settle, there will always be small bumps.

Even now, if I hit a really difficult patch in my life, then I might drink more than normal; but I recognise the situation and then can compassionately address the habit and bring things back into balance. Deeply ingrained unhelpful habits never go away completely even after you have got them to fade, so don't be surprised or upset if they resurface from time to time. When you are aware that old coping mechanisms can show up in difficult situations, you can avoid being sucked in to the old habits for too long and follow the new path that you created instead.

Life is hard and bad things happen, so also be realistic with your goals. Deciding that your eating will be what you consider to be balanced 100% of the time, and that old patterns won't ever emerge again, is absolutely not going to happen. So don't make that a goal! It is unrealistic and impractical. Instead, learn to ride the waves — learn from them and work to make them smaller. Any time you notice you are getting back into unhelpful habits, check in with yourself and revisit the plans you have made to help you get back on track.

Part 3

Happy and healthy – holistically

Chapter 6
The Wheel
of Wellbeing

Having introduced some tools for building a healthier relationship with food and reprogramming your unhelpful eating behaviours, it is time to look at another part of our journey together — helping you to improve all aspects of your wellbeing so you can be the happiest, healthiest version of you:

- The version of you that has plenty of energy to do the things you want to do, who has a clear mind and can make decisions that are aligned with your goals.

- The version of you that is able to deal with life's ups and downs and is able to pick yourself up after difficulties without needing to pretend you are okay when you're not.
- The version of you that feels good about yourself, and believes in yourself and what you are capable of.

To be this person, you need to look after yourself both inside and out. This means leaving a focus on the scales behind and instead looking after your body and your mind so you can function at your best and access the magic that lives within you; magic you might not even know is there!

The World Health Organization (WHO) sums things up very nicely with this definition of health:

'Health is a state of complete physical, mental and social well-being and not merely the absence of disease or infirmity.'

I love this definition because it is about **optimising health rather than just trying to avoid illness**. It has no focus on weight or size, but instead focuses on the good — building 'complete' wellbeing, which, as well as body and mind, takes into account the importance of relationships and human connection, our social wellbeing.

Being the happiest, healthiest version of you doesn't mean you'll never cry. Nor does it mean that bad things won't happen, or that you will no longer make mistakes in your life. Those things will still happen; they are all part of being human. What it does mean is that you will be better able to manage the tough patches, and work through things knowing there is a light at the end of the tunnel. It will also make it easier to maintain a healthy relationship with food.

This is about embracing the journey, too, rather than seeking a destination to arrive at and hoping you will just stay there. **Becoming the best version of you is a process you will continually need to work on, grow with and adapt to as your goals develop and your circumstances evolve.**

————

To help you work through this next stage of your journey, I want to introduce you to my Wheel of Wellbeing. This identifies the six key areas that I have found to be the most important to work on for my own physical, mental and social wellbeing. Over the coming chapters I will be taking you step by step through each of the segments of my Wheel of Wellbeing and sharing my top tips and tricks for making positive changes to your life in each area.

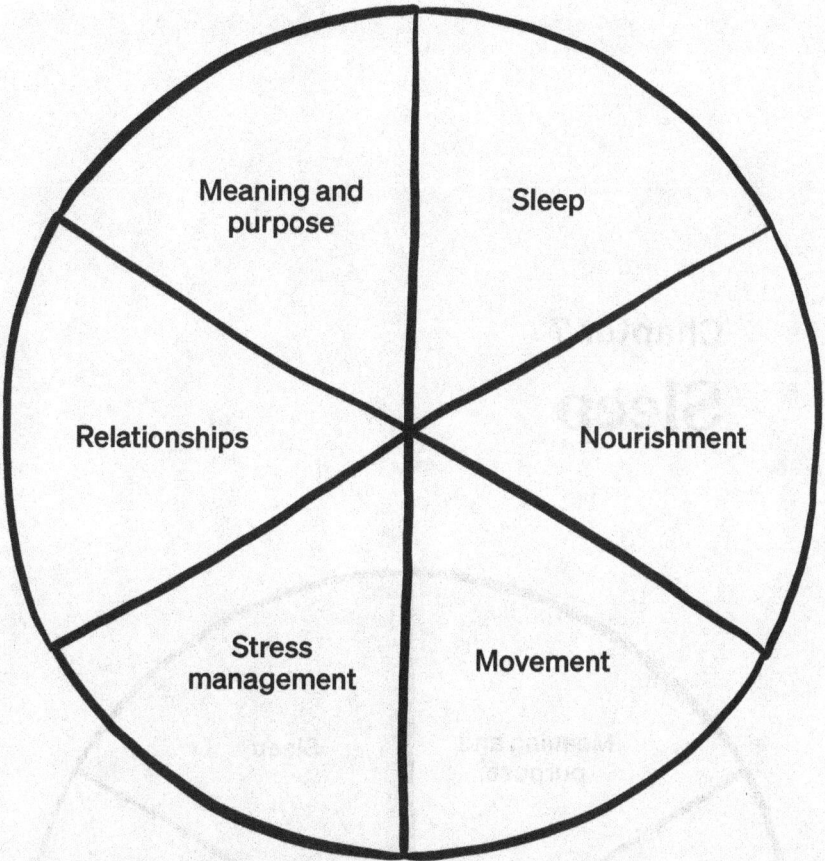

The Wheel of Wellbeing

- Meaning and purpose
- Sleep
- Relationships
- Nourishment
- Stress management
- Movement

Chapter 7
Sleep

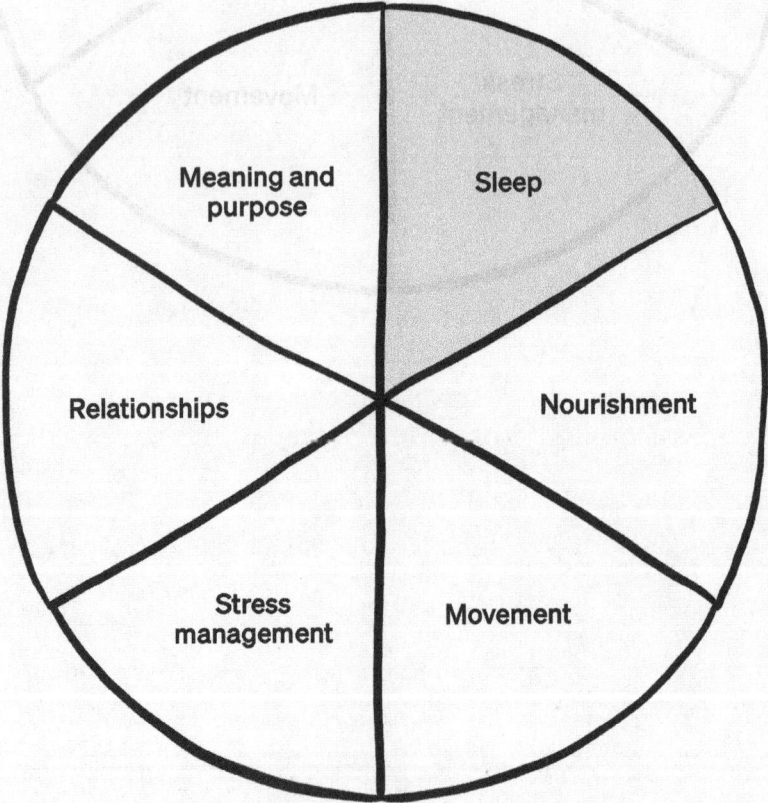

Meaning and purpose

Sleep

Relationships

Nourishment

Stress management

Movement

'Sleep is the golden chain that ties health and our bodies together.'

— English dramatist Thomas Dekker (1572–1632)

When it comes to improving your health and wellbeing, sleep is perhaps the most under-appreciated tool. Its impact on both your physical and your mental wellbeing is utterly profound — something I found out the hard way when my second child arrived in the world.

When my son Josh was just a couple of weeks old, his older brother, Zac, aged three at the time, had to have an operation to remove his adenoids and tonsils due to extreme sleep apnoea. In a haze of exhaustion after having been up half the night trying to feed Josh, my husband and I took Zac into the hospital to have his operation. My mum, who was over from the UK, stayed home to look after Josh.

While my husband tapped away on his keyboard in the waiting room, working, I slumped in a chair and closed my eyes, waiting for it all to be over.

We waited, and waited, and waited.

It was a 45-minute operation, yet three hours later, he still hadn't come out. Coming from a medical family, I knew things sometimes took longer than expected and was trying not to panic and ask questions every five minutes. Instead, I distracted myself and patiently tried to convince my husband that everything was fine.

But it wasn't. There were complications after the operation and Zac was unable to breathe on his own. After the medical team spent five hours trying to stabilise him, we ended up having to be transported in an ambulance, lights flashing, to Starship hospital where they had better facilities to look after him.

The weeks that followed were messy. My husband had to go back to work, so my mum ended up looking after Josh and working on him accepting a bottle while I slept at Starship with Zac, on a squab on the floor by his bed, intermittently trying to pump breastmilk which had to go into the hospital fridge ready for my mum to collect later in the day.

After lots more dramas and tense moments, we finally got home and my mum and I swapped places. She slept in Zac's room to keep an eye on him overnight, and I was back with Josh trying to work on his feeding — which wasn't going well.

I was beyond shattered.

A couple of days later, with Josh still waking up all the time and not sleeping well either during the day or at night, I started to have hallucinations. One night, I was apparently crawling on my hands and knees, crying and looking for Josh under my bed because I thought he was stuck under there. He wasn't even in the same room! As well as the nightly hallucinations, I also had so many deeply terrifying thoughts I was beside myself. I had experienced post-natal depression with Zac, but this was next-level.

A week or so passed and my mum had to go back to the UK. I remember being on the couch in our living room feeding Josh on a Monday afternoon and having that same terrible feeling I had had at age 19 when I had felt deeply unsafe in my own company.

But this time, I had a newborn baby in my arms.

Luckily, because of my previous experiences, I knew I needed to ask for help. I called my cousin Rachel, who was on her way to sit her midwifery exam, and said I needed her urgently. She skipped her exam and came to my rescue, for which I will be forever grateful. Rachel took me to the doctor as I was in too much of a mess to go on my own, and after a long wait the lovely GP I saw took the time to go through things properly with me. I was diagnosed with post-natal psychosis. The GP insisted I get three full nights of sleep immediately, and if I didn't commit to that and show her that I could get a plan in place, she said she would have to admit me to hospital.

Off I went home. My husband and Rachel sorted out the kids and Josh's feeding nightmares (which turned out to be severe lip and tongue tie), I put my ear plugs in and got my three nights' full sleep, and thankfully the hallucinations stopped. I felt terrible not being able to look after my newborn myself — that maternal instinct made it feel so wrong to step away — but I knew I had to do it both for him and for me.

This experience was the beginning of an utter fascination with sleep and just how incredible it is — and how torturous and dangerous it can be when you don't get enough! As well as my passion for nutrition and fitness, I became engrossed in studying sleep; something I still keep up to date with today. The more I learn, the more I am wowed by the magic of sleep and just how much it influences all our behaviours, including how we eat.

Sleep is so important and non-negotiable that I decided to make it the first segment of my Wheel of Wellbeing, because without it, all the other segments are harder to action.

What happens when we sleep?

Sleep allows your body to properly repair and replenish itself. When you sleep (typically overnight), an amazing clean-up happens in your body to get you ready for another day of wakefulness. Sleep is vital for a healthy immune system. It's when your short-term memory is converted into long-term memory. And, as I know all too well, it can have a profound impact on your mood. As someone who has been on and off antidepressant medication throughout my adult life, I know that without adequate sleep things can go south quickly on the mood front. Without sleep, you can literally lose your mind.

As I said in Chapter 4, sleep can also have a massive impact on your appetite because it increases the amount of the hormone ghrelin (which makes you feel hungrier) and at the same time decreases leptin (the hormone that gives you the message to stop eating). So fixing your sleep really is essential for your journey to create a healthier relationship with food. As well as making it a lot easier to make mindful and intentional choices, it helps you make nourishing choices, because (let's be honest) it is often the highly processed, salty, sugary foods that come calling when we are tired. Plus, adequate sleep also helps strengthen your willpower and boost your motivation, which again makes it easier to make choices that are aligned with your goals.

Sleep can also help improve your productivity, creativity and ability to solve problems. Having previously believed that to get the most out of a work day you need to put in as many hours as possible, what I have learnt about sleep has — spectacularly — proved me wrong on that front. **Making an impact and getting things done is about being effective and efficient,** as well as being able to do hard things when you need to, and nothing helps with that more than a good night's sleep. I get way more done in less time than I used to, thanks to good sleep, which gives me more time for other things in my life. Honestly, when you realise how good life can be when you are able to sleep well, you will never want to go back!

———

The official recommendation for sleep for adults is 7–9 hours each night — and that's time asleep, not just the time you spend in bed. If that sounds a long way from where you are now, panic not. I have lots of ideas and solutions to help you get there.

I never used to get that much sleep; I was a 'six black coffees a day, stay up as long as possible so I don't miss out on the fun' kind of person in my twenties and early thirties. But things are very different now, in my forties. I would be half dead if I lived like that these days! I now apply all the tools I know and do my utmost to get my 7–9 hours as often as possible, and it makes such a difference to my life. When I don't get enough good-quality sleep, I — like most other people who are tired — am short-tempered, snappy, drink more, eat more and am way less motivated to work, move or do . . . well, just about anything. That person is not the mother, friend, colleague, wife or version of myself that I want to be.

Along with using the smart tricks I will be teaching you about sleep, I have also had to make some changes to my expectations and to the expectations of others. To get enough sleep, it means there are things I have to say no to. I don't really get much time to myself in the evenings after the kids go to bed, and I am never really up with what is on Netflix. But for me, those compromises are worth it so I can function in a way that feels good and not like I am swimming against the tide every minute of the day, like I used to.

Humans are the only species on the planet who consciously choose to deprive themselves of sleep, which really is utter madness. This madness is reflected in the rates of mental health issues, obesity, diabetes, heart disease and other chronic diseases that are all made worse by sleep deprivation. **It is time for this to change.**

Sleep is a very active process. As you go through the night, you move through different stages of sleep. They include several stages of non-REM (non-rapid eye movement) sleep and REM (rapid eye movement) sleep.

In stage 1 of non-REM sleep, you are just dozing off; and then in stage 2, there is a slowing of the activity in your brain and body. Stages 3 and 4 are the deepest part of non-REM sleep — your body and muscles relax even more and your brain waves slow down. This deep sleep is believed to play an important role in body recuperation and effective thinking and memory.

You also have periods of REM sleep around the time you wake. REM sleep is when your brain activity picks up and most parts of your body, except your eyes and breathing muscles, experience temporary paralysis. This is the time when the most intense dreaming takes place. REM sleep is believed to be essential for your brain to consolidate new information and enhance your ability to learn and recall information.

Your sleep goes through 'cycles' that are approximately 90 minutes long. At the end of each cycle, you hit a phase of light sleep which it can be easy to be woken from. A pain, I know! (We will be talking about how to manage waking up on page 160.)

Historically, it was deep sleep that got all the praise and was focused on, but more recent evidence shows that REM sleep is equally important in its own way. Cutting your night short and skipping some of this dream state sleep can be very detrimental. Your body knows best, and there is a reason why our sleep was designed the way it is. We just need to get back in rhythm with it.

So how can we help you to get the 7–9 hours of sleep you need? What needs to change in your life to make this possible? I know it is not as easy as just getting into bed and turning off the lights! Sometimes it can be hard to fall asleep, right? And what about waking up in the middle of the night? And the dreaded mind-racing that can happen at 3 a.m.?

There are solutions, lots of them. It is possible to sleep well again!

How to get a better night's sleep

1. Get your light right

MORNING LIGHT

To fall asleep more easily at night, you need to take action in the morning! Humans are diurnal, meaning we have evolved to be awake during the daylight hours and asleep at night when it is dark.

But how does your body know the difference between day and night? And how does it make us feel sleepy at the right time? Well, your brain relies on light to figure this out.

Back in our hunter-gatherer days before artificial lights were invented, the process would have been simple. As the sun came up, our eyes would have been exposed to natural light. As the light entered the eye and hit the retina at the back, a message would have been sent up to a part of the brain called the suprachiasmatic nucleus. This is essentially like a central clock for your brain and regulates your circadian rhythm, your inbuilt roughly 24-hour cycle.

When your eyes are exposed to natural morning light, this basically kicks your body and all its systems into 'daytime mode', ready to get up and get moving! Critically, at the same time it also helps ensure that your body knows that in about 12–16 hours you are going to need to go to sleep again, and that the hormone melatonin will need to start rising to be ready for that time.

Nowadays, however, many of us don't get outside early enough in the morning, or for long enough, to get enough natural light on our eyes. And when we do go outside, it is now common practice to put sunglasses on even early in the morning, which is really unhelpful. Sunglasses are fantastic for when it is sunny and for sure during the daytime, but first thing in the morning they are not something you want to be wearing habitually.

Ideally, we would expose our eyes to natural light in the first hour or so of daylight, aiming for at least 10–20 minutes on a sunny morning or 20–30 minutes on a cloudier day. If you can't do that long, five minutes is still better than nothing at all. There is an added benefit to this, too: exposing your eyes to natural light also helps your body produce serotonin, the body's natural antidepressant, so there is a double win for making this part of your daily routine!

You might be thinking, *well, what about bright indoor lights in the morning, won't that do?* Not completely. If it is still dark outside when you wake up, it *is* a good idea to make your house as light as possible with artificial light initially, but that doesn't replace the need to go outside when it becomes light. Here is why. Your average indoor light bulb emits around 100 or so lux (a measurement of light intensity/brightness). Even on a cloudy day outdoors it is nearer 10,000 lux, and when it is sunny it's more like 100,000 lux. So, natural outdoor light is best for waking up your brain, even in the rain!

Getting natural light into your eyes can also help during the daytime. It is very normal to have an energy dip and feel sleepy in the afternoon; this is a natural part of your circadian rhythm. Unfortunately, though, in our modern world our workplaces don't often allow for this natural dip and we have to find a way to push through — which is commonly done with another cup of coffee or a bite of something sweet. However, if you can make it work with your day, get outside instead, even just for five or ten minutes. This can help suppress melatonin so you feel less tired.

As well as supporting your circadian rhythm, being outside in nature has other benefits. Research shows that people who spend more time in nature report feeling happier, calmer and having lower levels of poor mental health, in particular less depression and anxiety. If you can be active outdoors, you also get the benefits of exercise! Plus, you make vitamin D when your skin is exposed to sunlight, which is important for all sorts of things from keeping your bones healthy to supporting your immune system.

ACTION TIME! Put some of these tips into practice and see how they improve your sleep:

- Set an alarm or reminder on your phone to get you outside in the morning until that becomes a normal part of your routine.
- Eat your breakfast or have your first cuppa outside.
- Walk to a bus stop that is further away than your normal one to get additional time outside in the morning.
- If you are working from home, try taking a call outside in the morning, or do your first hour of work outside.
- If you are dropping kids off at school, park further away so you have a longer walk and more time to expose your eyes to natural light.

EVENING LIGHT

In the morning your eyes are not very sensitive to light, which is why you need lots of it to kick your brain into action. At night-time, however, the reverse is true. Your eyes become extremely sensitive to light and exposing them to artificial light can suppress the production of melatonin, making it harder to fall asleep!

Managing your light exposure both in the rooms you are in during the hours before bed and any additional light coming from screens, be it a TV, computer or mobile phone, can make a world of difference. I have noticed a huge improvement in my ability to fall asleep after we installed some dimmable lights in our house and started using lamps on low settings in the evenings rather than overhead lights. I am always reminded how powerful this simple step is when I stay with other people who keep lots of lights on in the house before bed. It is always much more difficult for me to get to sleep even when I have got over the 'new room, new bed' sleeping challenge. Dimming the lights in your house in the evenings is something I highly recommend. This is also super-helpful for kids if you struggle to get them to sleep.

When it comes to screens, I'm sure you know the deal — less exposure in the evening is better. On the odd occasion when I do watch TV at night, I change the settings and dim the screen; that's worth a try for you. With laptops and computers, go to the settings and change the screen to night mode, making it as dim as possible. The same goes for your mobile. Many phones, tablets and computers now have a timing option so they dim automatically at a time you choose. It is recommended that we try to avoid screens for at least an hour before bed, ideally more, even if they are dimmed. I know this is hard, but if you are struggling to get to sleep it really can help. It's a call you have to make based on your priorities.

These days, I keep anything I need to read on paper for the evening, and listen to audiobooks or podcasts rather than watching TV at that time. I know it's hard to avoid screens, with so much being accessible on devices now, so this is just about doing the best you can.

Another good idea is making it harder to pick up your mobile phone and just scroll away mindlessly, if that's a trap you fall into. I have a watch that links to my phone so I get a notification if anyone calls, which means I can leave my phone in another room — which means I check it less often. Super-helpful. Your willpower tends to be lower in the evening than in the morning, so don't rely on *that* to keep you on track. You need a plan!

When it comes to bedtime, make your room as dark as possible. For our early ancestors it would have been very dark at night — with no red lights on alarm sensors, no streetlights, no lights on in corridors. Make whatever changes are practical in your house to make things as dark as you can. Try dark or blackout curtains and having little plug-in sensor lights in the corridor (rather than leaving lights on) in case you need to get up in the night. Investing in a good eye mask is also something I highly recommend. The one I use is a complete blackout one (you can find it on my website) and it is an absolute game-changer! Even my husband, after vowing to never use something as 'girly' as an eye mask, now swears by his and wouldn't be without it. Some people also benefit from using ear plugs to block out noise.

2. Make time for sleep

Your body and brain don't understand the importance of responding to everything in your inbox late at night during the week. Nor do they understand the need to finish a TV series. What they do understand, and favour, is **consistency** and **predictability**. If you can keep your body and brain, most of the time, in the 24-hour circadian rhythm around which they have naturally evolved to function, you will be rewarded in many ways.

The more consistent you can be with the time you go to bed and the time you wake up, the easier it will be for your body to do what it needs to do. When you work with your body rather than against it, you are likely to find it will be easier to fall asleep in less time and you will wake up without always needing your alarm clock.

I know this poses challenges in our busy modern world, especially as some activities go on later into the evening than you would like. Sometimes you might need to wait up to make sure your teenagers get home safe from a party, and there will be dinners with friends where the connection with them is just as valuable for your mental wellbeing as getting enough sleep. This again is about doing the best you can, with where you are at. Most of us have at least a few things we can take control of and changes we can make so that we get to bed at a more consistent time *most of the time*. As I said before, sometimes we will have to make some sacrifices because we can't do it all and have it all — but it can be well worth doing that.

Getting up at a consistent time is also something to work on, even at the weekend. This doesn't mean you can't sit in bed chilling and enjoying a cuppa on a Sunday morning, but if you are regularly feeling like you need to 'catch up' on sleep at the weekend, lying in will only work against you trying to get your body into a good cycle.

If you are always feeling like you need to catch up on sleep, always need your alarm to wake up and never feel fully ready to get out of bed when it's time, you are not getting enough good-quality sleep. I recommend that you look at the other ideas in this book to help you address your sleep on a day-to-day basis so you don't have to function like this anymore.

WORKING WITH YOUR CHRONOTYPE

Something else that can make it easier to fall asleep and wake up more easily is seeing if there is anything you can do to live more in line with your natural chronotype. This is your body's natural, inbuilt desire to want to be awake or asleep at different times of the day. It is the pattern you would naturally fall into if you were not working, had no commitments or responsibilities, were away from all technology and reminders of what the 'time' is, and were left to your own devices for a while without needing to conform to a certain pattern. Many of us don't often get the chance to experience this, unless perhaps we are camping. But if you did this experiment, where do you reckon you would fit? Would you be a morning type? An evening type? Or somewhere in the middle? Under 'Sleep' in the resources section on page 295 there's a link to an online questionnaire on this — give it a try.

It is suggested that having different chronotypes served as a survival advantage in our earlier hunter-gatherer days — it meant that not everyone was asleep at the same time, so there was a smaller window of risk of being attacked or having your area invaded. It is predicted that around a third of people fit into morning types, a third are neutral and a third are evening types — so whichever type you are, you are not alone!

In a way our modern world is cruel, in that it highly favours morning types rather than evening types. It can be really challenging if you fit into the latter category. Hopefully, as sleep gets talked about more and more, workplaces might finally become more flexible at supporting people to work in line with their natural rhythms — knowing that work outcomes are likely to be better.

If you do feel like you naturally tip one way or the other with your chronotype, there are things you can do to take advantage of this. I am a morning type so always work out in the morning, do my heavy-brain-load activities first thing and organise any meetings for the afternoon. This is easier for me because I am self-employed, but think about whether there is anything in your life that you could do to make things work better for you. If you are an evening type, is there any way you could arrange to work later, when you are more productive, and get up a bit later in the morning? I understand that this might be impractical, but even having more people around you who understand our natural biological variance might make them more supportive of things you struggle with in our morning-skewed world.

3. Get the temperature right

For you to be able to fall sleep and stay asleep, your body and brain need to cool down by almost 1 degree Celsius (1°C), which is why it is always easier to fall asleep in a room that is too cold than one that is too hot. It is also the reason why, if you have kids or grandkids, you might find they keep kicking off their sheets or hanging their legs and arms out of the bed even after you have tucked them in for the tenth time. Their bodies are just trying to cool down.

To help cool your body before bed, something I find works really well is having a warm bath or shower. While this warms the outside of your body up at the time, when you get out it can make it easier for your core body temperature to drop down to where it needs to be for sleep.

Room temperature matters, too. The optimal temperature for sleep is 16–20°C, with 18°C being the average I aim for. This is much easier to achieve in winter than in summer, particularly in the North Island of New Zealand and many parts of Australia. But again, as with all of the tools I suggest using, this is about doing the best you can with the resources you have.

In winter, I personally avoid having a heater on in our bedroom and no longer use an electric blanket. As I live in New Zealand's South Island, where it gets really cold overnight for much of the winter months, I do sometimes use a hot-water bottle for my feet. There is usually residual heat in the house from the fire, but I allow our bedroom to feel cold.

In summer, I do my best to keep our house cool by opening the windows and blinds early in the morning and then closing them in the afternoon, like they do in Europe, to keep the heat out. The best solution for you to keep your house cool will depend on where you live and the options you have available to cool your house or apartment.

Something I highly recommend, however, is tinting your windows if your house gets hot in summer. I wish I had known about this sooner when we were living in Auckland. We got tinted film put on the windows of our bedrooms, and immediately it stopped the rooms getting up to 30+ degrees at night! They were still around 20+ degrees — still a bit too hot but infinitely better than before! Google 'window tinting' and you will find all sorts of companies who can help.

4. Manage your busy mind

Honestly, there is nothing more annoying when your head hits the pillow than being bombarded with an overwhelming number of thoughts whizzing around your brain.

Why did she look at me that way? Maybe I offended her? . . . How am I ever going to get to that meeting tomorrow when I only have 20 minutes to travel, parking will be a nightmare and there are all those road works on? . . . Did I feed the cat this morning? Oh, there is still washing in the machine, I think! I can't be bothered, it will just have to go smelly; I'm too tired. Why don't other people in this house do more and help out? No one sees how much I do . . . I really don't want to go to that dinner tomorrow. Why did I say yes? I always do that; always say yes to things I don't want to do. What is *wrong* with me, why can't I just say no? Is that the police helicopter again? I'd better check the local Facebook page to see what's going on . . .

Sound familiar?

Despite this being really annoying, it is a very normal thing to happen when, for the first time that day, you actually sit (well, lie) still. Your brain goes into overdrive trying to process and deal with all the noise and data input it has had all day.

The worst part is that there is often a negative skew to the chatter in your head. Do you ever lie in bed thinking, *I did really well in that presentation today. I am so proud of how I handled that difficult conversation. That dinner I made tonight was just top-notch.* Not often. Your brain has a negative bias, so is far more likely to focus on the bad rather than the good. Historically, this negative bias would have served as a survival advantage — it would have been far more important to remember information about where the tiger was approaching from rather than about the pretty flowers you passed on your daily hunting mission. These days, however, this negative skew is not as advantageous. While it is, of course, helpful to be across problems and be aware of potential dangers, it is also vital that we are able to notice the good and foster thinking that encourages positive emotions to support good mental wellbeing.

Put into practice, this means that we have to catch ourselves ruminating on the bad and rewire our thinking to focus on the good. This can be done through the practice of mindfulness and meditation. There are lots of incredible resources available to help you with this. I am personally a big fan of the Calm app, but I know that Headspace and Insight Timer are very popular, too.

As well as practising mindfulness and meditation, there are a few other tricks I use to calm my mind before bed. One is a journal; I write things down that are going round and round in my head, because once the thoughts are captured on paper the swirling often stops. I do this in the kitchen or the lounge before bed, rather than in the bedroom, to stop me associating this 'download' of mess from my head with the room I sleep in.

There are other things to keep out of your bedroom to avoid associations which can lead to wakefulness. This includes a TV, your laptop, your tablet and ideally your phone. Go back to an old-school alarm clock, or use an old phone that doesn't have any apps or Wi-Fi. It really does make a difference. Having devices that are connected to the 'outside world' in the room where you sleep causes what is called anticipatory anxiety, which is anxiety that is based on the feeling you might be needed at any moment, or you might be 'missing out', or something is about to happen. This can compromise the quality of your sleep as your brain is getting the message that it isn't safe to be deeply asleep because you might need to act imminently. Think about what it feels like when you need to catch a flight or meet at a certain time for a job interview, or something else you know you can't miss. You almost never sleep properly beforehand; your brain knows what is going on!

Associations can be positive, too. You might have a certain smell that you associate with sleep. Or, by lighting a candle, doing a quick–slow massage of your feet or hands, or listening to the same music again and again before bed, your brain will start to connect those activities with sleep, which can be supportive.

5. Manage caffeine and alcohol intake

When it comes to sleep, what you drink and when you drink it matters. Particularly with caffeine and alcohol.

Firstly, let's look at caffeine. As you probably already know, caffeine is a stimulant. That means it can help you feel more awake — which sounds like a good thing, right? And sometimes it can be! There are, however, a couple of problems with it, especially when you have too much.

Caffeine has a long half-life, which means it breaks down slowly in your body. If you have your first caffeinated drink at 7 a.m., about half the amount of caffeine will still be circulating in your system 5–6 hours later, and a quarter of that caffeine will be going round 10–12 hours later, between 5 and 7 p.m. Before bed and while you sleep, there will still be some caffeine hanging around. And that is with just one drink. What about the next one you have mid-morning, the one after lunch and even the one before bed?

The caffeine circulating in your system may or may not stop you going to sleep. Some people can indeed go to sleep easily at night after having consumed a lot of caffeine during the day, but even if that is you, it doesn't mean the caffeine hasn't affected your sleep. It will have. Caffeine circulating in your system while you are sleeping reduces the amount of deep non-REM sleep you are able to achieve. This can mean you are more likely to wake up not feeling refreshed and needing another caffeinated drink (or three). A vicious cycle.

Another thing to understand about caffeine is one of the ways it makes you feel less tired. During the day your brain naturally builds up a chemical called adenosine. As the adenosine level rises, it links to special receptor sites in your brain and creates what is known as 'sleep pressure', which is, essentially, the desire to sleep. Under ideal circumstances, adenosine is high at night before you go to bed so that you feel sleepy. Combined with high levels of melatonin, which you'll have if your circadian rhythm is on track, this means you will be ready for sleep and will fall asleep without too much trouble.

Caffeine interferes with this process. It blocks the adenosine receptor sites in your brain and makes you feel less tired. Which sounds good, until it is not. The adenosine that isn't able to link to a receptor site just builds up in your brain until the caffeine has finally run out, then — *BAM* — rebound tiredness kicks in. You get a dump of adenosine hitting your brain that makes you feel unreasonably tired and in need of — you guessed it — something to perk you up! Coffee, anyone?

Too much caffeine can also increase feelings of anxiety, something I personally have become very aware of. I can just about tolerate the caffeine in two cups of tea a day, but give me a double-shot coffee and I will be a blithering mess! Of course, we are all different when it comes to caffeine and our sensitivity. Some people are more sensitive than others, but when it comes to sleep, less is still best!

The last thing to be aware of is that you can become tolerant to caffeine. This means that over time you need to have more to get the same energy-boosting hit, and then more and then more. Not ideal, especially if you have anxiety or sleep issues in the mix.

It isn't all doom and gloom, though. There are some great things about caffeinated tea and coffee, which contain antioxidants. What are antioxidants? Without trying to make things too complicated, essentially they help fight 'free radicals' in the body which can cause harm if their levels become too high. Free radicals are linked to multiple health issues such as diabetes, heart disease and cancer.

Also on the upside, because it is possible to clear caffeine from your system as long as you don't have too much and you drink it earlier in the day, you can enjoy caffeinated drinks without compromising your sleep too much. Current recommendations are that adults should have less than 400 mg a day, and less than 200 mg a day if you are pregnant. Personally I would encourage you to aim as low as possible for your daily baseline, say 200 mg a day, and then if and when you need the odd pick-me-up after a late night or when working on a big deadline you can have that extra caffeine you need to get you through and it will be effective as a stimulant.

To help guide your choices, the table on the following page shows how much caffeine is in different drinks . . .

Drink	Amount of caffeine
Drinking chocolate (250 ml)	5 mg
Decaf long black (130 ml)	19 mg
Green tea (250 ml)	31 mg
Cola-type soft drink (355 ml can)	35 mg
Black tea (250 ml, average brew)	47 mg
Instant coffee (250 ml, medium strength)	51 mg
Plunger coffee (250 ml, average brew)	66 mg
Coffee (cappuccino) (260 ml)	105 mg
Energy drink (500 ml bottle)	160 mg

Data adapted from Ministry of Health, *Eating and Activity Guidelines for Adults, 2020.*

As a side note, a 50 g bar of chocolate contains the same amount of caffeine as a can of cola; so if you're having chocolate late at night you might find it negatively impacts your sleep.

———

The second drink to deal with regarding sleep, and your wellbeing in general for that matter, is alcohol. This one is even harder for me to manage than caffeine, but alcohol can stop you getting good-quality deep sleep in much the same way caffeine can. Sadly, there is no amount of alcohol that is 'okay' when it comes to sleep. Less simply is best and, like caffeine, the closer it is to your bedtime, the bigger the impact on your sleep.

Alcohol is also a carcinogen, which means it increases your risk of cancer, and it causes all sorts of other health issues. However, before you shut this book right here and think, *Claire, this was going so well until now, I don't like what you're saying!* hear me out.

It is about finding a balance that works. In all of the 'Blue Zones' in the world — the places where you find the highest percentage of people aged 100 and older — some form of alcohol exists within their culture and is enjoyed by their people. But *not* in excess, *not* all the time, and most often as part of social occasions with other people. In these areas of the world, the negative effects of alcohol are probably offset by other factors that we know encourage people to thrive. Blue Zone cultures have food patterns based on whole foods, and the people are typically highly physically active, have a strong sense of community, are connected, and have purpose and a positive outlook. The way they consume alcohol is very different to the way that it is often consumed in our society where 'too much, too often' is a common trend and drinking is a common way to de-stress, disconnect from work or try to connect with other people.

If you don't drink much, or at all, then this will be no big deal. If, however, you feel like alcohol could be a problem for you and you drink more than you want to or know is good for you, then this is a good time to reflect on what is driving your drinking. Return to the awareness and reflection steps on pages 101–108 and think about what role alcohol is playing in your life.

It is also useful to reflect on how alcohol affects your eating. If you have ever drunk alcohol, you will know that it can stimulate your appetite and, just like when you're tired, it can increase your craving for salty foods. I know that with my friends a bag of chips can be demolished in under a minute once the cocktail maker has been shaken and the drinks sipped. If alcohol is indeed playing into your challenges with food, it is well worth considering how you can reduce the amount and frequency that you are drinking. Going through my four-step process in Chapter 5 will help with this.

In New Zealand there are government guidelines for keeping alcohol consumption low. To be clear, these don't mean 'no risk';

they mean 'lower risk', with less always being best. Here are those guidelines:

- At least two alcohol-free days a week.
- On days that you drink, women should have no more than two standard drinks, men three.
- Over a week, the upper limit is drinking no more than ten standard drinks a week for women, 15 for men.

A 'standard drink' is the amount of drink that contains 10 g of pure alcohol. This is 330 ml of 4% beer, or 100 ml of 12% wine, or 30 ml of 42% spirit. For more details, head to www. alcohol.org.nz.

With alcohol, any steps in the direction of 'less' will be helpful for you in many ways. It comes down to your priorities and what works for you and your life.

6. Manage night waking

There are few things more frustrating than lying in bed staring at the ceiling in the middle of the night, knowing that you want to be asleep, and *need* to be asleep, but you just can't seem to get yourself to drift off again.

There are *some* things that aren't in your control when it comes to night-time waking, like getting older, or the impact of certain medications, but there are several things you *can* do, so there is good news here!

Firstly, I recommend working on the basics I mentioned earlier, including having a regular bedtime, wearing a good eye mask and ear plugs, as well as managing caffeine and alcohol intake. Those can certainly help to get night waking sorted.

Beyond that, one of the most important things to do is to remove all the clock faces from your bedroom.

Why? Because if you are in the habit of waking up at night, what is one of the first things you do when you wake? Check the time, right? As well as the light on your phone, watch or clock not helping your chances of falling back to sleep, checking the time kickstarts an internal conversation about what that time means.

Oh no . . . It's 2.45 a.m.! I *always* wake up at 2.45 a.m. What is *wrong* with me? It has been months like this now. I have to get up in three hours . . .

I'll be too tired to go to the gym . . . How can I get fit if I can't get to the gym? And it is so expensive, too. Maybe I should text Sarah now and say I can't go to the spin class so she knows?

And I'll be so tired, I'll spend another day eating too much . . . And work — I have *so* much to do tomorrow. I hate having this sleep problem . . .

. . . And now it is 4.03 a.m.! How am I still awake?

As long as you have an alarm, ideally an old-school one as I previously suggested, and you know it will wake you up when you need to be up, **you do not need to know the time in the middle of the night**. Give this a try for at least a fortnight, and see for yourself if this makes a difference. It has worked so well for me.

The second thing to do is avoid staying in bed too long if you are just lying there awake. This creates an association between *bed* and *wakefulness* and *anxiety around sleeping*. Instead, if you feel like you aren't going to fall back asleep easily, then get up. Go into another room with lights as dim as possible, and read, listen to some very calming music, a meditation or an audiobook — and then, when you are sleepy again, return to bed.

My third tip is to replace counting sheep (which the research shows doesn't really work) with doing a 'mental walkthrough' in your mind. This basically means slowly going through in your mind, step by step, a process you do all the time, or a walk you go on, in the highest possible detail. For me, I run through my day. My alarm goes off, I get out of bed, I walk to the bathroom. I open the cupboard. I pick up a flannel. I walk to the sink. I turn on the tap. I wet the cloth. I wash my face. I turn off the tap. I hang up the flannel to dry. I walk to the towel hanging up. I dry my face . . . and so it goes on.

Instead of running through your day, it could be how you cook a meal, how you do the washing, or a walk that you often do, but always slowly, really really slowly, going through the process step by step. This should be calming. If it is not calming, move on; try something else. Different things work for different people.

––––––––––

If you have tried all of the strategies I've suggested here and still aren't able to sleep properly, it really is worth seeking professional advice. Sleep specialists can do some amazing things to help you reprogram your sleeping, and these won't necessarily need to involve any medication. If you have been to your GP or a sleep specialist before, you will no doubt have experienced how reluctant they are to prescribe sleeping medication, especially in the long term. Many of the drugs used really just act as sedatives instead of supporting the normal, healthy process of sleep. As with many things, the best fix really isn't a pill.

It is also worth considering if perimenopause or menopause is affecting your sleep. The average age for menopause (which means you have not had a period for 12 months) is 51; perimenopause is the phase of life leading up to that, and normally lasts between seven and ten years. As well as lifestyle changes, it might be that menopause hormone therapy (MHT), previously known as hormone replacement therapy (HRT), might be helpful for you.

I started MHT last year, when I turned 42, because my sleep quality had started to decline despite making all the lifestyle adjustments possible. I was also having debilitating brain fog, memory issues, anxiety and crazy pins and needles, all of which started within the year before without me changing anything I was doing! For me personally, MHT has changed my life.

If you, too, are in your early forties and struggling with the many symptoms of perimenopause but were thinking you were too young for MHT, think again. It might work for you. You will need to seek advice from a GP who is across women's health, because time and time again I have seen women struggling so much but they have been told by their GP to come back when they are having hot sweats. This is not the current evidence-based advice, so if that's what you have been told, then seek a second opinion. You shouldn't have to feel like you have to suffer in silence.

For more on this topic, see 'Perimenopause/menopause' in the resources section on page 296.

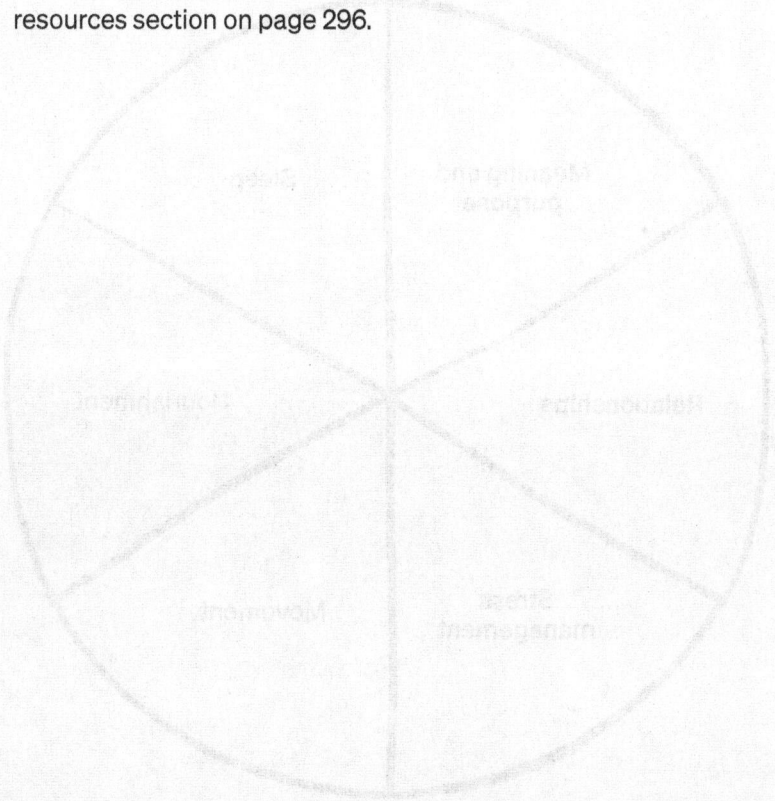

Chapter 8
Nourishment

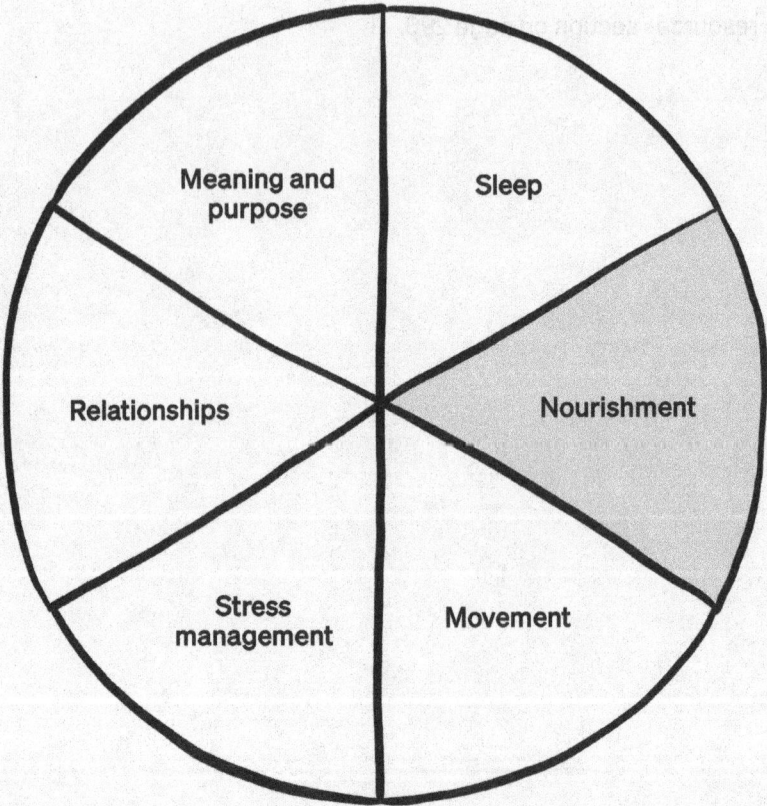

What you eat makes a big difference to how you feel and how well your body functions, but working out what to eat is the complicated part, right?

Type 'what to eat to be healthy' into Google and you will find over 3 billion pages of tips, guidelines and suggestions. Some information is consistent, much is not.

'What to eat to lose weight' is another common search. This one serves up 2.4 billion pages filled with even more confusion: YouTube videos about reducing belly fat, lists of foods to avoid, 'superfood' recommendations, meal plans and a mishmash of other such conflicting information.

Why has it become so hard to work out what to eat?

Differing opinions, confusing messages and impossible-to-understand food marketing all play their part. Doctors disagree with each other, as do seemingly credible nutrition experts and personal trainers — and that's before you take into consideration the snippets of advice given to you by family, friends, colleagues and people you follow on social media!

How to navigate the nutrition advice minefield

The study of nutrition is relatively new compared with other areas of science, and, like any other topic of research, new findings are being discovered all the time. For example, early research indicated that cholesterol in foods had impacts on the cholesterol levels in your body, and subsequently there were official recommendations in government guidelines about limiting foods that are high in cholesterol, such as eggs and prawns. However, as more research was done, it was discovered that this impact wasn't as big as had first been thought, and so the recommendations around cholesterol have changed; eggs and prawns are no longer being limited for most people. So one of the confusing things is that **even with credible nutrition advice, things genuinely change!**

Ideally, new research would be considered in conjunction with all of the other information that exists. The quality of the new research, any biases and any study limitations need to be considered, and if advice is given subsequently it needs to reflect the best summary of the evidence in that space. This is something that registered dietitians and registered nutritionists, who are accountable to a professional board, are obligated to do. Even so, professional experience and personal biases can still play a role regarding the advice given. So even within a group of registered nutrition professionals there will be some degree of variation in focus.

Alongside registered dietitians and nutritionists are the many people who call themselves nutritionists but whose study and experience can vary massively! Some have done years upon years of study in areas such as medical herbalism and naturopathy, which is an approach that some feel works for them; others, however, might have done next to no study at all. At the moment, anyone can call themselves a nutritionist without having any formal qualifications. You really can't compare the advice given by someone who has done a 14-week online course in nutrition to that from someone who has studied full-time for five years.

While it is fantastic that so many people now have an interest in nutrition and are looking to upskill themselves, it is really important for you — the person on the receiving end of their advice — to be **mindful of the potential limitations**. This is particularly important if the advice encourages a dieting mindset, like needing to track every gram of food you eat, cutting out entire food groups or being really restrictive. Do also be mindful that anyone can cherry-pick through the research, cite other wellbeing gurus they follow or refer to compelling podcasts to back up their points of view. In my experience, the more opinionated someone is that their way is 'right' and everything else is wrong, the less they often know about the true science of nutrition (which simply is not black and white).

Health professionals other than registered dietitians and nutritionists — namely GPs and pharmacists — are often a first port of call for nutrition advice. However, do be aware that they may have very limited professional nutrition training: unless nutrition is a personal interest of theirs which they have chosen to study, their expertise may be limited. The reason I say this is because at Mission Nutrition we frequently get calls from people who have been given the advice to go 'sugar-free', 'no-carbs' or to 'cut out gluten and dairy' after a trip to the doctor, and 99% of the time this isn't the right approach when we review their history.

Next comes the frequent advice on nutrition that appears on TV and radio, which often ends up being sound-bites of information that showcase mixed opinions. Being a voice in the media myself, I know how hard it can be to ensure that the right balance of information comes across in my interviews. In all written media, I ask that I can check my quotes before they publish, and I make sure I ask about the other people being interviewed on the topic to ensure that my comments land as they should do alongside the other voices. However, this is certainly not common practice with people who are interviewed. So be aware: **what you read is often a filtered version of the truth**.

Live TV can make it easier to present balanced information, but sound-bites in the news can be a real challenge — even the images used alongside your comments can change the meaning of the few words you were saying. Again, question what you watch; don't simply accept it as truth. Documentaries in the food and nutrition space also warrant a closer look at the validity of some of the claims and recommendations they make. There are some fantastic research-based programmes that are really helpful, but alongside these there are some really rogue ones. They can be really fancy productions, may be very one-sided and focus on fearmongering, encouraging you to give up entire food groups. Also bear in mind *where* a documentary is set. There are some seriously dodgy things being covered up by the food industry in certain parts of the world, particularly the US. You shouldn't watch a documentary based on American food issues and think that everything that is said there is relevant here in New Zealand — much of it is not. Also, some 'documentaries' are more sensationalised than factual, as well as not being particularly relevant for us. **Be aware of what you take from what you watch.** Check who is behind the show and who paid for it, and question what their motivation might be.

Magazines often showcase nutrition advice in the form of meal plans, 'healthy recipes' and 'top tips to get you ready for summer', but, as you will know, this advice is often conflicting and, except for magazines like *Healthy Food Guide*, is often not written by a health professional. Its credibility needs to be questioned.

Then there is social media — which is like the Wild West when it comes to nutrition advice! *Anyone* is free to offer their opinion and advice in this space, and it can be so hard to avoid getting sucked in, especially with those before and after photos, compelling stories and people with huge followings who look how, in your mind, you have always wanted to look. A recent study from researchers at Deakin University's Institute for Physical Activity and Nutrition looked at nearly 700 Instagram posts by influencers and brands with more than 100,000 followers, and found that 45% — nearly half — contained inaccurate nutrition information! As I have mentioned before, be really mindful of who you follow and the messages you get drawn into in this space.

Finally, while there will be snippets of great advice that you receive from other people, please always stop briefly and question the information. While some less conventional things can work sometimes and are possibly worth considering, you do need to make sure that you aren't being led into a dieting mindset or causing harm to yourself in some way.

The bigger picture

Given all the conflicting information about nutrition, alongside the complex language used — like 'micronutrients' and 'phytonutrients' and 'bioavailability' and 'phytoestrogens' — I fully appreciate how easy it is to feel completely lost and not know where to start.

So, let's take a step back, start at the beginning and consider the bigger picture.

It is estimated that our species, *Homo sapiens*, has been on the planet for around 150,000–200,000 years, originating in Africa. Back then, as you can imagine, food sources were very different and life spans much shorter. As early humans spread throughout the world over the centuries that followed, food sources would have changed depending on the country they were living in.

Over time, living in different parts of the world, humans learnt to adapt to different ways of eating depending on what was available in each place. There would have been certain foods which supported survival, and others which, when missed out on, would have compromised bodily functions. As our brains evolved, we started making tools to make hunting easier, and started cooking food — which made it safer, tastier and, although we didn't know it then, made some nutrients from the food easier to absorb. Humans went on to domesticate animals and learnt how to grow their own food to supplement their hunting-and-gathering efforts, which was a helpful step towards establishing a reliable supply of food.

For most of human history, our food supply has been based on whole, minimally processed food, which is what our bodies have evolved to process. Fast-forward in time through to modern farming, and developments in food processing, production and transporting of different foods from one part of the world to another, and things are very different.

My mum, who is now in her seventies, grew up on a farm without a fridge until she was 16. The only processed food they bought regularly was canned fruit and, on special occasions, cornflakes. Cakes, biscuits, jams and marmalade were all homemade. They did have puddings, but the portions were small and the ingredients simple.

I am in my early forties, and when I was growing up there was definitely more commercially processed food around — Mars bars in the school tuck shop and an array of processed breakfast cereals and packet noodles — but I only recall eating this type of food maybe 5–10% of the time, max. When you compare this with how much processed food the average family buys now, the mind boggles! A 2019 University of Auckland report titled 'State of the food supply' estimated that almost 70% of the packaged food sold in our supermarkets is considered to be 'ultra processed'. A 2021 study from the University of Otago found that around half the energy intake of kids came from ultra-processed foods. How crazy is that?

While this change might not feel dramatic to you if you are aged 50 or under, it really is extreme when you look at how we have been eating for most of our history. If 150,000 years was equal to 24 hours, then 70 years would be equal to 1.68 seconds. That is the fraction of evolutionary time that human beings have been eating commercially processed food.

The development of mass food production has undoubtably had some incredible benefits. The ability to freeze and can food has meant many foods are now available in some form all year round. Frozen and canned veges make it very easy for people to eat nutritious food in a cost-effective way. Cooking and preserving food can help ensure it is safe to eat, and (for example) steaming and rolling oats helps them cook more quickly so they become a realistic option for breakfast.

There is, of course, a massive downside that comes with the ability to commercially process food. These days, far too much of our food supply is so far removed from its original form that it is, quite honestly, frightening. And because it has become so 'normal' to eat processed food, many people don't realise what a problem it can be when it is eaten in large quantities.

The rise in technology and sophisticated processes in food manufacturing mean that we now have foods which hijack our brain's reward pathways and so are very difficult to stop eating. Tell yourself you will just have a handful of those cheesy nachos, then suddenly the whole bag is gone? Salted caramel chocolate and ice cream just disappear when they're in your house? The taste, texture, crunch and smell of highly processed foods have been cleverly designed to overcome any amount of willpower!

When fat and sugar, or fat and salt, or sugar and salt — or all three — are combined together, it is very hard for your brain to say 'no more, thanks' because this combination can override your body's fullness signals. They're not natural combinations — in nature, no food exists that has these three things combined in the way they are in many processed foods, especially foods that hold very little nutritional value.

With whole foods, it is much easier to trust your fullness signals and manage the amount you eat. There are only so many avocados, apples or plain unsalted nuts, for example, you could eat on their own in one go. Even when combined in something like a bowl of homemade chicken, vegetable and barley soup, there is still only so much you can eat before your fullness signals kick in. One reason for this is that whole foods require you to chew. This slows down your eating and gives leptin time to send its signals to your brain. Unfortunately, we have become very accustomed to eating food that is blended up or broken down in such a way that some of the work our body expects — and actually benefits from — is taken away.

Research published in the journal *Cell Metabolism* in 2019 showed that when people were asked to eat either whole foods or highly processed foods, those who ate the highly processed foods on average had to consume 500 more calories each day to feel equally satisfied. That is mind-blowing.

Variety also overrides our fullness signals and encourages us to eat more. If you had, for example, a box of chocolates that was all the same flavour, evidence suggests that you would likely eat a couple less in one sitting compared with a variety box. Why? Because we experience something called flavour fatigue — you essentially get bored with the same flavour, which encourages you to stop eating.

––––––

If you are struggling to manage the amount you eat, really take a moment to soak these things in.

It is now so normal for many of the everyday foods we eat to be so highly processed that our brains don't register them as real food. Even some of the less processed, simpler treats like salted caramel chocolate or really good-quality ice cream have combinations of nutrients that make it hard to stop eating them. It can be difficult to really honour our fullness signals when these foods are a regular part of our life.

However, despite the amount of processed food that exists in our modern world and the damage that alcohol can do, you will know by now that I strongly believe **it is not helpful to label any food or drink as 'good' or 'bad'**, because it always comes down to context.

These are words I avoid saying at all costs to my children.

If you enjoy a bar of chocolate mindfully once a week, is that bad? No.

What about a dessert with your friends at the weekend while enjoying a delicious home-cooked meal, laughing and sharing stories? Also not 'bad'.

I like to think about food and drinks being on a continuum. At one end are nutrient-packed whole foods which are minimally processed and help our bodies to function at their best and feel good. At the other end are foods that we don't need to survive, ultra-processed foods and drinks that lack nutritional value but are fine when enjoyed occasionally, without guilt.

On the following page is a visual representation of this continuum, which I feel is a helpful framework to consider. It is very hard to clearly define what fits into each category — things like bread, muesli bars and cereals are not all created equal, after all. The pictures here are just examples of an overall theme, not an exhaustive list of all foods that fit into these groups, so don't get bogged down in the detail.

The foods on the left of the continuum are unprocessed or minimally processed and have high nutritional value. These are great when planning your meals; this is where to focus your attention. Equally, including some of the processed foods in the next section along can be helpful — these also have high nutritional value.

It is hard to put numbers on this, because there is so much variation in the different types of food, but my recommendation is that if around 80–90% of what you are eating fits into the first two sections most of the time, you are on to a winner. And variety is key to maximise your opportunity to get the balance of nutrients your body needs to function at its best. Coming up, I will be sharing my top tips and tricks to help make it easier for you to make these foods part of your everyday life.

Unprocessed or minimally processed foods with very high nutritional value	Processed foods with high nutritional value	More highly processed foods with moderate nutritional value	Ultra-processed foods or foods with very little nutritional value
Foods that are in their natural form or close to it. One ingredient or no ingredients list is needed on the label. Fresh, dry or frozen vegetables, fruit, grains like brown rice, quinoa and oats, legumes, meat, fish, seafood, eggs, nuts/seeds.	Foods with minimal ingredients on the food label. Dried fruit, canned fruit, olive oil, milk, cheese, unsweetened yoghurt, canned fish, canned pulses, tempeh/tofu, quorn, canned tomatoes/vegetables, dense wholegrain traditional-style bread, muesli, seed crackers.	Processed breakfast cereals, muesli bars, wholemeal bread/wraps, crackers, vegetarian sausages/processed protein alternatives, sweetened yoghurt.	Sugar-sweetened beverages, sweet and savoury packaged snacks, reconstituted meat products, packaged frozen meals, highly processed chicken nuggets, ice cream.

→ Increasing level of processing and reduced nutritional value

174

Some foods are more highly processed but still have some nutritional benefits and can be useful when you have a busy lifestyle. These are foods that fit somewhere around the third section of the continuum. For example, I occasionally use wraps, canned chilli beans or pre-crumbed fish on a Friday night and have low-fibre crackers at the weekend with some blue cheese. Bear in mind that within this group some options are more nutritious than others. Some cereals are much closer to candy than they are to brown rice, and all processed breads aren't created equal.

Finally, the foods and drinks in the right-hand section sort of speak for themselves: they are things our body doesn't need to function. But this doesn't mean that you can never have them, or that you need to feel bad about eating them. This is putting them in their place and working to enjoy them **mindfully and intentionally** rather than eating them out of habit or to manage difficult emotions (as we discussed on pages 92–99).

For myself, I can easily pass on the sugary drinks and have no desire to buy bakery items at the supermarket or a hotdog at a soccer game — these just aren't my thing. But if there is crème brûlée on the menu on the odd occasion that I go out to eat these days, I am all in. I also really love jam, especially our homemade gooseberry one with corn crackers or a slice of cheese. Marmalade, too — old English. Yum. Both are high in sugar, but they taste really nice and eating them occasionally is something that gives me joy. The same goes for gelato, which I adore. We don't have it at home because it would be far too hard for me not to eat it every night, but a few times a year, often over summer, I come across a gelato shop which has flavours that are a 10 out of 10 for me and I will order some and thoroughly enjoy eating it without feeling any guilt at all.

To live a long and fulfilling life that feels good, you don't need to be 100% sugar-free or never eat foods that you love! Banishing all the treats you enjoy is likely to only make you crave them more.

KEY MESSAGE

KEY MESSAGE

Perfect eating is the enemy of healthy eating.

What makes your 10–20% list?

So if around 80–90% of the foods you eat are from the first two sections on my continuum (the ones that are highly nutritious), that leaves room for 10–20% of other foods. There are two ways I decide what goes into my 10–20%. One is what really helps the convenience of my life and therefore gives me more time to spend with my kids and more opportunities to sleep. And the other is what I *really* enjoy — the things that hit 8 or 9 out of 10 in terms of how good they taste.

For me, convenience-wise, this is fresh filled pasta, vege sausages, vanilla yoghurt, nut bars, the crumbed frozen fish fillets and wraps I mentioned earlier, and a few other things.

For the stuff I really enjoy occasionally, kettle-style salt and vinegar chips. A really good custard square with thick icing. British Maltesers (yes they are *very* different to the ones we have here, which for me are easy to bypass). Really good kūmara fries.

ACTION TIME! As you start to become more mindful about what you eat, you will notice a gap forming between you thinking about eating and you actually eating. It is this gap that can change your life. It is the opportunity for you to become intentional about your decisions — you can think, *what is it that I really want to eat?* Is it a cake, cookie, slice, pizza, burger, chips? Are these 9 out of 10 that you will *really* enjoy? Or are they more like a 4 out of 10 that might be best to pass on because they just aren't that good?

Putting the 'nourish' into nourishment: how to get enough of the stuff that makes you feel good

If you have committed to trying to improve the nutritional balance of what you eat before, most likely there will have been some degree of restriction involved. There was probably a list you were given (or created for yourself) of all the things you needed to remove or not have as part of a healthier way of eating.

I get that this might seem logical, but in practice it is super-unhelpful because it focuses your brain on deprivation and gives a negative skew to what you are trying to do. Instead, **the approach I encourage is focusing on adding in more of the foods that help your body work at its best and help you feel your best**. Whole, minimally processed food. In this approach, you essentially crowd out foods that aren't as nourishing for your body, rather than stop eating them altogether.

KEY MESSAGE

Focus on addition, not subtraction.

When you start eating more whole, minimally processed foods overall, you will find that you are giving your body more of the nutrients it needs to function at its best. You will find you have more energy, your bowels function better, it is easier to manage food cravings, it is easier to eat to your natural appetite signals, and you will want less of the highly processed foods.

This approach will also help you create a much more positive mindset around food, which is very necessary. After all, you are human — you need to eat to live, and you sure as heck should enjoy it!

Here are the foods to focus on **adding in** to make the good things happen ...

Veges

The first thing to focus on is adding in more veges. When I finally gave myself permission to eat more food, after having restricted what I ate for years, I found that dramatically increasing the amount of vegetables I was eating had an extraordinary effect. Now that veges are a big part of what I eat every day, I have never felt as good, and I have never found it easier to make choices about other foods.

Here are just a handful of the benefits of veges:

- They are packed with fibre, which helps support a healthy digestive system and better bowel motions — the value of which isn't to be underestimated! Have you ever been constipated? Not a nice experience, is it?
- Research suggests that having plenty of veges can help reduce your risk of depression and anxiety and also assists with the management of these challenges.
- With the vast array of vitamins, minerals, antioxidants, phytonutrients and other goodies that vegetables contain, they help keep your heart and brain healthy as well.

All the other organs and systems in your body are kept in good working order, too. Vegetables are foods we evolved to eat!

- When you eat vegetables in their whole form, rather than blended down or turned into powder, they require you to chew, which is more important than you might realise! As I mentioned earlier, chewing slows down your eating and gives you time to realise you are full.
- Vegetables that are lower in carbs have a high water and fibre content, which makes them quite low in energy. This means you can eat lots of them and that high volume can help with satiety (feelings of fullness).

For more on the impact of nutrition on mental health, check out Professor Julia Rucklidge from the University of Canterbury, who does some excellent work in this space.

SO, HOW MUCH VEG TO AIM FOR?

My recommendation is 5–6+ servings of veges a day. A serving is around a handful — ½ cup cooked, canned or frozen veg, or 1 cup of green leafy veges, or one medium-sized tomato.

When it comes to fruit, two servings is a good guide (again, a serving is about a handful), occasionally three for those who are more active. Now and then I might eat four servings of fruit. There are also days when I only have one or two serves of veges. Don't get too hung up on things — this is about what you do **most of the time,** remember!

These 5–6+ handfuls of vegetables are the less starchy, lower-carbohydrate ones; they don't include potato, kūmara, taro, yams or green bananas, which I pop alongside the other carbohydrate-containing foods as you will see a bit later. Remember: there is nothing wrong with potatoes and the other starchier vegetables. It's just that they are best considered separately from the less starchy vegetables because *nutrition-wise* they aren't quite the same. Vegetables with a higher carbohydrate component are more energy-dense (have more kilojoules) than those with less starch and more water. A cup of cooked potato provides between three and four times the energy of a cup of cooked broccoli, for example. I'm not encouraging you to start looking up the calories or kilojoules of your veges by raising this — that is a habit best left in the '80s. I am just trying to highlight how different two things which are both classified as vegetables can be!

The non-starchy veges you're looking at to make up your 5–6+ are things like broccoli, beetroot, carrots, lettuce or kale, cabbages of all types, cucumber, tomato, peas, etc. I suggest you aim for a wide variety of veges overall — enjoying all the different colours as each has their own unique combination of nutrients.

ACTION TIME! To get 5–6+ handfuls of veges most days, this is what I do. Have a look at these and see which ones could work for you.

First, at two of my meals each day, which for me is lunch and dinner, I aim to have 2–3 handfuls of vegetables. This is around half my plate (or the equivalent if it is something like soup or a casserole where all the veges are mixed in).

- For lunch in the summer, I make salad veges the base — whatever is in season and therefore affordable. Things like lettuce, cucumber, tomato, grated carrot, grated courgette, spinach, capsicum, mushrooms, bean sprouts, fennel, snow peas, beetroot, onion and green beans.
- When salad vegetables get more expensive or I have run out of things I have grown, I start making my own coleslaw. I buy a whole cabbage and shred up about a quarter or a half a week, depending on the size, and store it in a container in the fridge lined with damp paper towels to stop it going

dry. I often add some chopped herbs such as parsley and mint. I then do the same with 3–4 large carrots: wash and grate them and put them in a separate container, this time with dry paper towels. Each day, I grab a handful from each container and make that the base of my lunch, adding protein, healthy fat and some form of carbohydrate. Storing the base veges separately makes them last much longer!

- At the weekend I like to roast up a batch of veges, whatever I can find on special, along with odds and ends left over in the fridge. I then keep the roasted veges in the fridge and enjoy them as part of a salad.
- In the cooler months I get into soups and veg-loaded casseroles with plenty of pulses for protein and extra fibre. A cheap way to have a healthy lunch! As I travel a lot for work, I put this in my portable food pod which keeps it hot for up to six hours — definitely something worth trying! Check out where to get these pods on my website.
- Omelettes are also a winner for a light meal and are my go-to on busy nights. I use about two handfuls of veges and two eggs per person. Onion (white, red or spring), mushrooms, tomatoes, leafy greens (try frozen free-flow spinach), capsicum and courgette all work super-well — you can even add peas (with a little chopped mint . . . so good!).
- With any mince dish, like casseroles, curries, risotto, lasagne, etc., I find a way to add as much veg as I can. When I make a bolognese-type sauce, for example, I use two onions instead of one, and add grated carrots, courgettes or mushrooms (sometimes all three!). I'll use two cans of tomatoes rather than one, and often add lentils to make the mince go further and add extra fibre.
- I add extra grated or chopped vegetables into almost everything I cook. After an excess of courgettes last

summer, I found ways to put them in practically *everything*. One thing that worked really well was mixing grated courgette through rice just before serving. It softens slightly and really is delicious! I do it all the time now — give it a go.

- If I am having crackers for lunch and tomatoes are in season, that will be what I have on top along with some avocado or hummus. I will also have some extra chopped veg on the side or some soup to get to two serves — most of the time, anyway; nothing is ever 100% of the time!

- I don't really eat sandwiches or wraps because I never ate them growing up, but they're useful for lunch on the run. Here it's about cramming in as much veg as you possibly can and having extra veg on the side.

- When we have burgers at home with the kids, I use a lettuce wrap rather than a bun — you need a sturdy leaf like iceberg or cos lettuce (also very easy to grow) so it doesn't just fall apart and spread cheese, gherkins and sauce everywhere! You can do the same with falafels, meatballs and lamb koftas to get those extra veges in there. However, if I'm out, say in a pub after a day's skiing or hiking, and fancy a burger, then I'll just go for the bun, chips and all, and really enjoy every bit of it. It's all about balance.

- Mix up your mash. I am a big fan of a 50:50 mix of potato and cauliflower (when it is in season); such a great way to get an extra serve of a low-starch vege. Smashing peas or broccoli in with your mash is also a good option, as is the combo of carrot, parsnip and potato.

- If I am eating out and want more veges in my meal, I sometimes order an entrée and two sides of vegetables to have as my main. This is a really helpful strategy if you eat out a lot, as vegetables can be very light on some main-meal menus.

Once I have my lunch and dinner meals sorted, I am often 4–5 handfuls into my goal of 5–6+. Now I just aim for at least one additional serving. Sometimes I have this with my breakfast — mushrooms or spinach with some scrambled eggs at the weekends, or a veg-packed smoothie. Other times I have it as a snack at some point during the day, which for me is often mid-afternoon. This could be carrot sticks or cucumber with hummus or cottage cheese, or a ripe tomato if they're in season.

When it comes to smoothies, you will see from the recipes on my website that I look to keep them to a maximum of one serving of fruit plus the veg and some form of protein. I have an awesome green smoothie recipe with spinach, a carrot smoothie with (you guessed it) carrots, and a red velvet one with beetroot. All well worth trying. The reason I stick to one serving of fruit is that once the food is in a blended form you don't get the benefit of chewing it, so it can be really easy to take in more fruit than you want or need.

Juices are worth a mention, too. Veg-only juices with a base of high-water veg (like celery, cucumber or lettuce) can be a helpful way to add an additional nutrition boost, though you still need your whole vegetables to provide the goodness of the fibre in them! Juicing fruit, however, just concentrates the sugar and the end product has far less nutrition than it might seem. Having fruit juice very occasionally is fine but it's not something I would recommend doing every week.

⸻

To make all this affordable, know that **frozen veges are fine** — and sometimes better than fresh, especially if the fresh ones have been stored for some time. Also, to maximise the nutrition you are getting from your veges, either steam or bake them rather than boiling them in lots of water.

One final note: to ensure my kids have enough veges in *their* day, they get veges in their lunchboxes, veges at dinner and sometimes veges as snacks. At our house we also have a 'veg-only' policy before dinner — if the kids are hanging around the kitchen telling me how hungry they are, they can help themselves from the veg box, packet of frozen peas or any other veges they can find. It works a treat because there is never, ever another option for them. They have simply learnt to accept it.

Power up on protein

Protein-rich foods provide the building blocks (amino acids) that your body needs to repair tissues, grow and function properly. Protein also helps you feel full after eating and less likely to pick and nibble half an hour later. Evidence suggests that if your meals or snacks are low in protein, your brain will encourage you to keep eating in order to try to get enough protein. Fascinating stuff!

Focusing on having enough protein in each of my meals (and any snacks I have) has been one of the most helpful things I have done to curb my cravings and make healthy food choices. It has become a foundational part of how I plan my meals day in and day out. I love that by focusing on eating more of the things that make you feel good and feel naturally full, you end up wanting less of the foods that *don't* make you feel great without even having to try! This is a mindset to embrace.

Protein is found in a variety of different foods, so there is something for everyone.

- Animal sources include meat, fish, seafood, chicken, eggs and dairy products. Animal proteins contain all 9 of the 20 amino acids that are considered to be 'essential' — meaning that your body is unable to make those amino acids itself so you have to get them from food. Animal proteins are also generally higher in nutrients like iron and vitamin B_{12} than plant proteins are.

- Some plant sources, such as quinoa, hemp seeds, chia seeds, edamame beans and soy products like tofu or tempeh also contain all 9 essential amino acids.
- Other plant sources, such as pulses, nuts and seeds (except hemp and chia) don't contain all of those essential amino acids, but provided you have adequate amounts of a variety of plant proteins you will be able to get what your body needs. They are often good sources of fibre and, in the case of nuts and seeds, a fantastic way to get healthy fats.

One thing to be mindful of is the increasing number of highly processed plant-based foods on the market, many of which have long ingredients lists and are by no means considered whole foods. So, while those are great and convenient sometimes — and I use them myself — they do fit into the third section along the nutritional value continuum on page 174.

HOW MUCH PROTEIN DO WE NEED?

In this book, as far as possible I am trying to give the broader picture when it comes to how to feed our bodies, but two areas where I do feel it is really useful to have some awareness of specific numbers are protein (see below) and fibre (coming up on page 190).

So, bear with me — and keep the bigger picture in mind as those numbers come out here.

Current nutrition guidelines suggest aiming for 78–130 g of protein a day for an average adult. Let's be clear, though: in real life there is no such thing as an 'average' adult! As we are all so different, this is just a starting point; a range to consider. (Also, note that if you do a lot of exercise you might need more protein again.)

On a practical, day-to-day basis — without the need to count every gram — this guideline means you are looking for around 20–25 g of protein at each of your main meals; around 10–15 g if you are having a snack. If you are more active, it might be up to 30 g per meal or even a bit more, along with higher-protein snacks. If you don't generally snack, you might need a bit more protein in each of your meals.

To add context here, on the opposite page I've given the protein content of some common foods. Again, don't get too hung up on the exact numbers, as they can sometimes vary from brand to brand — just look at the trend. Some foods are clearly higher in protein than others. And, you don't *have* to just eat meat and eggs! If what you eat is varied, all the smaller amounts of protein in those foods add up. As you can see, you even get protein from pasta and peas!

HOW MUCH PROTEIN IS IN THAT?

To be honest, I don't always hit the target amount of protein every day — and that is okay. Once again, it is *most days* that matters. Like you, there will be some days when I have a handful of muesli on the go for breakfast, grab some sushi for lunch and then default to eggs on toast for dinner, because life happens. **Let go of the judgement or expectations that are too high.**

The reason I encourage you to have enough protein most days is simply that, in my experience, it can be really helpful when you are looking to improve your overall nutrition, particularly because of its ability to help you feel fuller for longer.

ACTION TIME! As there is no 'one size fits all', I encourage you to experiment with your meals and find what works *for you*. You might find that getting a good 15 g at a meal really helps you feel full for much longer than at the moment; or you might need nearer 20 g or 30 g to get to this place. Trust yourself and your body. You know

Plant-based proteins		Animal-based proteins	
Tofu (small block; 170 g)	21 g	Canned tuna (95 g)	24 g
Baked beans (½ large can)	11 g	Chicken breast (uncooked, 100 g)	23 g
Chickpeas (1 cup/175 g)	11 g	Beef steak (uncooked, 100 g)	22 g
Shelled edamame (½ cup/75 g)	10 g	Salmon (uncooked, 100 g)	20 g
Soy milk (250 ml)	10 g	Hoki (uncooked, 100 g)	15 g
Grainy bread (2 slices)	8 g	Eggs (2 medium)	11 g
Dried pasta (75 g)	7 g	Mussels (shelled, ¼ cup/62 g)	11 g
Cooked quinoa (1 cup)	7 g	Cheese (2 slices/40 g)	11 g
Raw mixed nuts (handful/30 g)	6 g	Plain yoghurt (200 g)	10 g
Rolled oats (½ cup)	5 g	Cow's milk (250 ml)	9 g
Green peas (½ cup)	4 g	Medium latte (300 ml)	9 g
Peanut butter (1 tbsp)	4 g	Cottage cheese (2 tbsp)	4 g
Corn cob (½ cob/100 g)	4 g		
Almond milk (250 ml)	2 g		
Sunflower seeds (1 tbsp)	1 g		

yourself better than anyone else, so have a try and take note of what works for your life.

Know that when you get the hang of roughly how much protein is in different foods, you won't need to focus so much on the numbers — that is just an initial step to help increase your awareness in this space. For personalised advice on this, my team at Mission Nutrition can help.

GETTING ENOUGH PROTEIN IN YOUR MEALS

It's easier to get enough protein in some meals than it is in others. Breakfast is the one people often struggle with (including me), unless you are having eggs. But a good first step is just to start having more protein in your meals and snacks than you are at the moment, if you are currently nowhere near the recommended range. This way there's no need to get obsessive and add a whole other problem that you don't need!

Remember that alongside what you might consider the 'main' sources of protein — meat, fish, eggs, dairy and so on — you will also be getting some protein from things like bread, pasta, corn, peas and suchlike, and it all adds up over the day.

Be mindful to focus on variety, and not default to thinking you just need to eat more meat to hit the targets. Fish and seafood are a really great way to get more protein. Fresh, frozen and canned fish are all good options, as well as mussels, which are not only super-affordable but also amazing nutrition-wise, with fantastic amounts of iron, zinc and omega-3 fats! Having mussels every week would be ideal.

Eggs are also brilliant, and within a balanced eating plan you don't need to limit them unless you have heart disease or are at risk of heart disease, which includes people with type 2 diabetes.

Pulses are a really affordable way to add more protein and fibre into your everyday meals. I add them to all my soups, mince dishes and casseroles, as well as salads. Swapping rice or pasta for quinoa is another great trick to increase protein.

What about protein powder? These are powdered-down and concentrated proteins from various food sources, such as milk (whey proteins), grains, peas or seeds. Most people can get all the protein they need from real food. However, protein powders are very convenient if you are busy and sometimes struggle to eat enough protein each day, particularly if you are very active.

Carbs to suit you

When it comes to nutrition, there is nothing more controversial than the topic of carbs, and with the rise in popularity of keto and other low-carb diets and the accompanying demonisation of things like bread and pasta, it is hard to know what advice to follow.

So here's the thing.

First up, there is no 'one size fits all' when it comes to carbs. Also, what suits you in your twenties might be different from what suits you in your thirties, and different again when you hit your perimenopausal/menopausal years. Those years are when there is an increased likelihood of developing insulin resistance as a result of all the hormonal changes going on during this crazy phase of life. If you're like me, and currently in this stage, you might find it helpful to have a bit less carbohydrate than you used to. There also might be phases of your life when you are more active and need more carbs, and seasons when you are more sedentary and need less. **It is all about finding the balance that works for you at the time!**

Secondly, not all foods classified as carbohydrates are created equal. Highly processed supermarket bread is not the same as a wholegrain sourdough made with the traditional fermentation method. Oats, brown rice and potatoes are not the same as processed breakfast cereals, cereal bars and chips. So let's not tarnish them by association. Also, some protein-rich foods which have huge nutritional benefits, such as pulses and quinoa, also contain carbohydrates. Consequently, avoiding them just doesn't make sense. The exception to this is if you have gut issues like IBS and need to limit pulses to help manage your symptoms.

Over the years, I have done a lot of experimenting with changing the amount of carbohydrates I eat, and it has been super-interesting. When I don't have enough I find I don't sleep as well, and I tend to feel hungry even when I have eaten enough protein.

Not having enough carbohydrates is also unhelpful in the bowel department. Carbohydrate-rich foods can be a great source of both soluble and insoluble fibre; the amount of each type of fibre depends on the food. We need 28–38 g of fibre a day for good health and to reduce our risk of bowel cancer, but on average we only get around 20 g. So, being aware of how much fibre there is in food really matters.

The table opposite shows how much fibre is in different foods, broken down by the type of meal you might eat them at.

GETTING CARBS RIGHT FOR YOU

While not having enough carbs causes me problems, if I have too much then I don't feel good either! So I have worked to find my sweet spot. I have some carbs at each of my meals, mostly the minimally processed type and probably a quarter or a third of what I am eating overall at that meal. Sometimes I have a bit less and sometimes a bit more (and it is definitely more the week before my period — it is *very* normal to feel hungrier then, so adjusting your food to allow for that is okay!).

I am sharing this with you because rather than me telling you 'This is how much you need to eat', I would love you to be your own experiment and see what works for *you* and makes *you* feel good. Give yourself permission to try different things and see how you feel. Having said that, both professionally and personally, I wouldn't recommend keto or a similar super-low-carb approach unless there is good reason. Keto is used for managing epilepsy that is non-responsive to treatment, plus a handful of other medical conditions. Outside of that, a **moderate** approach that focuses on good-quality carbs with an amount that is tailored to *you* is my suggestion. Especially since some sources of carbohydrate are valuable sources of soluble and insoluble fibre as well as resistant starch, which is important for healthy bowel function and can help reduce the risk of bowel cancer.

	Food	Fibre content
Breakfast	Banana (1 medium)	2 g
	Weet-Bix (2 bricks)	3.5 g
	Wholegrain cereal (¾ cup)	6 g
	Wholegrain oats (½ cup)	6 g
	Frozen berries (½ cup)	4 g
	Baked beans (½ cup)	7 g
	Chia seeds (1 tbsp)	5.5 g
	Soy-linseed bread (2 slices)	5.5 g
Lunch	Salad greens (1 cup)	1 g
	Avocado (¼ medium)	2 g
	Mixed seeds (2 tbsp)	2 g
	Wholemeal wrap (1)	2.5 g
	Vita-Weat 9 Grains (4 crackers)	3 g
	Ryvita (2 crackers)	3 g
	Pear (1 medium)	4 g
	Four-bean mix (¼ cup)	7 g
Dinner	Potato, skin on (135 g)	2.5 g
	Kūmara, skin on (135 g)	2.6 g
	Brown rice, cooked (1 cup)	3 g
	Quinoa, cooked (1 cup)	4 g
	Lentils, cooked (½ cup)	3.5 g
	Chickpeas, cooked (½ cup)	6 g
	Vegetables, cooked (1 cup)	3.5 g
	Wholemeal pasta, cooked (1 cup)	6 g

Continued...

	Food	Fibre content
Snacks	Carrot and celery sticks (1 cup)	2.5 g
	Hummus (3 tbsp)	3 g
	Whole almonds (20)	3 g
	Peanut butter (1 tbsp)	3 g
	Plain popcorn (2 cups)	3 g
	Apple (1 medium)	3.5 g
	Dried figs (2)	4.5 g

BEYOND BREAD

Looking for ideas other than wholegrain bread to get your carbs in? Try these!

Brown rice, quinoa, oats, barley, bulghur wheat, lentils, chickpeas, black beans, kidney beans, potato, kūmara, taro, green bananas, whole fruit, wholegrain crackers, home-popped corn kernels.

One of today's challenges is that many of our standard meals are carb-focused, and often include a lot of highly processed carbs. Cereal and toast for breakfast, sandwiches for lunch, a muesli bar for a snack and a good serving of spuds, rice, pasta along with some protein and veges for dinner. This can work for some people, but if you find that moderating the amount of carbohydrate works better for you, some suggestions follow to help make that happen. These also help you get more veg and more protein. Check them out and see which ones will work for you.

BREAKFAST

- Rather than a bowl of muesli, a splash of milk and maybe a spoonful of yoghurt, try switching things around. Have a bowl of unsweetened yoghurt along with a serving of fruit and a sprinkle of muesli with some additional nuts and seeds. Less carbs, more protein, and healthy fat, too. A win.

- If you are normally an egg-on-toast person, see whether one piece of toast works with a couple of eggs, or two thinner slices with some veges on the side and some healthy fat from a slice of avocado.

- If you like porridge, try stirring a handful of frozen berries in at the end. And using milk rather than water will ensure you get more protein. If you add a dollop of peanut butter or some nuts and seeds on top, this will add even more protein along with healthy fat. Some people find that a scoop of protein powder in the mix helps if they get hungry not long after eating porridge . . . everyone is different! If you add extras to your porridge, you could then use a slightly smaller portion of oats which will help tip the overall balance of this breakfast and could keep you fuller for longer.

- If you are an overnight oats fan, add in plenty of chia seeds and make it with milk and yoghurt to boost the protein and, again, moderate the amount of carbs you have here.

LUNCH

- Lunch bowls are a great way to get heaps of veges, along with a good amount of protein and carbs to suit you. This is pretty much my go-to lunch at least 4–5 days a week: two handfuls of veges, about 20–25 g of protein, some carbs and a little healthy fat.

- With soups, we often default to having a couple of slices of toast alongside. You might want to see how just one slice suits if you have more pulses and plenty of protein in your soup to make you feel fuller. Or try making a soup that is a complete meal, such as chicken and barley soup which has everything you need in it (veg, protein, fibre-rich carbs), and leave the bread out altogether.
- Frittatas are a fantastic lunch option that can include plenty of veges, including a few starchy ones like kūmara and pumpkin. And being made with eggs, they are a naturally easy way to get protein. Serve with some wholegrain crackers and avocado or peanut butter if you want some crunch as well as healthy fat in the mix, too.
- A sandwich made with a dense, wholegrain bread with some protein like tuna, chicken, egg or hummus and heaps of veges inside as well as on the side is an easy go-to lunch option if you are a bread fan.

DINNER

- 99% of the time I have some carbs with my dinner, around a quarter of my plate. To get a nice full plate that works for me overall, I also need two handfuls of veges and enough protein to make me feel full. If you think that, like me, a more moderate approach to carbs would suit you better, don't feel that it has to be an 'all or nothing' thing. You could have a small potato or two at dinner, or a few spoonfuls of rice or pasta. Work out what suits *you*. If you have no carbs and then end up eating biscuits after dinner, what have you achieved? Not much. It would have been better if you had given yourself permission to have some carbs with your dinner.

Feel-good fats

Another endless debate that could take up an entire book on its own is the one around fat. But again, it all comes down to context.

In a nutshell, **fat is not to be feared**. Fat is essential to keep our cell walls healthy and maximise the absorption of the fat-soluble vitamins A, D, E and K, as well as fat-soluble antioxidants like lycopene and beta-carotene. It is also essential for supplying the body with omega-3 and omega-6 essential fatty acids which (like essential amino acids) the body cannot make itself. Fat can also be used as a fuel source for the body.

However, fat is a very energy-dense nutrient compared with carbs and protein. So how much oil you splash in the pan or how much butter you spread on your toast needs to be considered in balance with the other foods you are eating. For example, a tablespoon of oil has the same amount of energy as a slice of bread or a large banana. This is not a 'bad' thing — I mention it only so you can see how the different things you eat in a day can add up.

When it comes to oils, I recommend choosing the best quality that you can afford. Cold-pressed is definitely worth opting for over more highly refined oils if you can make that work within your budget. I choose cold-pressed extra virgin olive oil for most uses — salad dressings, when I make homemade chips and when I am cooking on a stovetop. Avocado oil can be used in the same way as olive oil, but as it is more expensive I mostly use it where I can enjoy the taste, such as in a salad dressing. For a stir-fry or Asian-style cooking, I tend to use sesame oil or peanut oil.

When I need an oil that has a milder flavour, like for baking, I tend to use cold-pressed rapeseed (canola oil) — this is much higher quality than standard canola oil or other similar vegetable oils. I very occasionally use coconut oil when I am making curry, but mostly I use it on my skin!

Some of the stars when it comes to healthy fats are nuts and seeds. I have two Brazil nuts every single morning to get my daily dose of selenium, something we often fall short of in this country. Selenium is a powerful antioxidant which protects our body against damage, helping regulate blood pressure and keeping our immune system healthy. Where I can I add a sprinkle of seeds to a meal, aiming for a couple of tablespoons of nuts/seeds a day consistently. If you have nuts in your pantry, do be aware that it is easy to grab endless handfuls for a snack. I stick mostly to unsalted nuts because it is very hard to stop eating the salted ones!

Avocado is another shining star which I have most days when it's in season, either as a spread or in a salad. As well as being high in heart-healthy fats, it contains a surprising amount of fibre.

When it comes to butter, which (like most people) I love, I do have a little, mostly when I am making scrambled eggs. When I bake, I use recipes that work with one of my favourite oils, to boost the amount of unsaturated fats in there.

If you have high cholesterol, then a plant sterol spread may be helpful. Otherwise, if like me you eat mostly whole foods and not a lot of processed food that is high in saturated fat (like cookies, cakes and pastry), having a little butter is fine. Again, it is about context and balance.

Hydration

Looking at what we need to focus on **adding in**, for many of us drinking more water is a helpful goal.

The body of an average-sized adult contains about 35–45 litres of water, which is around 60% of their body weight. Our bodies need water for key processes like digestion, absorption, transporting food, removing waste and controlling our temperature (thermoregulation). It's not surprising that inadequate hydration can cause problems like tiredness, constipation, poor concentration and headaches.

So how much water do you need?

While 6–8 glasses or 2–3 litres a day is a recommendation you might hear — and is a good rough guide — the exact amount you need to drink varies from person to person. The amount you need is affected by things like your age, your gender, how active you are and how much time you spend inside and outside.

The rule of thumb is to drink enough to make sure that during the day you are passing large volumes of very pale straw-coloured pee. If it is dark, you aren't drinking enough. (The exception to this is if you are taking B vitamins, which can make your urine a fluoro yellow shade! The colour of your pee can't be relied on here, so keeping to 2–3 litres is a good place to start.)

The amount you need to drink does include milk, tea, coffee and so on as well as water, but do keep in mind the impact that caffeinated drinks have on your sleep. In my opinion, water is the best and first choice.

Here are some tips to keep yourself well hydrated during the day:

- Create a new habit around times to drink water. For example, when you first wake up, when you need a break from your emails, when your phone rings, or before each new task. Schedule alarms to remind you if need be.
- Fill up a large water bottle or two in the morning and take it with you for the day.
- Consider getting a water bottle with a trackable gauge, so you can see how much water you've had and by what time of the day. For a cheaper option, use a permanent marker

to mark lines on a transparent water bottle.

- If you're beginning to feel the onset of any of the signs of dehydration I listed earlier, your first port of call should be to get yourself a drink of water.

It is also important to know that you *can* drink too much water. You might have heard of the lady who died after she drank four bottles of water in 20 minutes while sweating heavily. Drinking so much in a short space of time put her electrolytes out of balance, causing her brain to swell. It is best to spread what you drink throughout the day. If you sweat really heavily or do a large amount of high-intensity exercise, then electrolyte replacement drinks may be appropriate. We can offer personalised advice on this at Mission Nutrition.

How *when* you eat affects your health

While tuning in to your hunger and fullness signals is a super-helpful tool, there is one thing to be mindful of. For most of human history, eating mostly happened in the daylight hours. When light bulbs became widely available in the early 1900s, this changed the pattern of our days significantly. In a nutshell, it is not a natural thing for us to pick and nibble all day, or to start eating at the crack of dawn and still be eating late into the night.

If you are currently in a routine like this, your body will have become accustomed to this pattern of eating. Because the hormone ghrelin can be released in anticipation of a time when you normally eat, your body may genuinely send you hunger signals as late as 9 or 10 p.m. at night.

This is where the use of the hunger and fullness tool needs to be balanced with what we know about the inbuilt 24-hour circadian rhythm we humans have. For adults, research indicates that (much like our ancestors) eating within an 8- to 12-hour window, ideally during the daylight hours, can be beneficial for our health. Current research shows an improvement in liver, gut and brain health, as well as mood and cognitive function; and symptoms of reflux can also reduce.

There isn't enough evidence to suggest a need to go below 8 hours, however, as it can be hard to meet your nutritional needs in this short time. Also, it starts to become impractical and has negative impacts on relationships if you no longer eat with other people, so this is not something I would recommend. For more information on research into the timing of eating, check out Professor Satchin Panda from the Salk Institute for Biological Studies, who is one of the world's leading experts in this area.

I have been keeping my eating (mostly) within a 12-hour window, usually around 10 hours, for the past three years and I have found this incredibly helpful. Breakfast for me is around 9.30ish (though I get up quite a bit earlier) and I have dinner with my family around 6.30 or 7 p.m. In the evening I drink herbal tea.

Once again, this is a **most of the time** pattern for me — there is always flexibility. When I go out to dinner with friends I eat later, and if I have a super-early start to work I will eat a bit earlier that day.

ACTION TIME! Figuring out when you should eat is something to experiment with and, once again, find what works for *you*. It is not about becoming super-rigid or it being a rule where you feel you can either pass or fail. Instead, it is an opportunity to tune in to how it feels to eat in a different pattern from how you do right now, and to notice whether (and how) your hunger and fullness signals change when you do this. If you currently eat late at night and manage to get out of that routine by shifting more of your nutrition to the daylight hours, you might find you sleep better, too!

Making nourishing choices the easy option

If you have food in the fridge when you get home from work, is it easier or harder to make a nourishing evening meal compared with going to the supermarket after you leave work and thinking about what to cook? It is much easier if you have food already in, right? And easier again if you have a plan about what you are going to cook!

What about choosing a topping for your crackers at lunchtime? If you are in a bit of a rush, and jam is at the front of the fridge and an avocado right at the back of the vege drawer underneath everything else, which topping do you end up going for? The jam, probably. Because it is EASIER.

When we are time-poor and life is busy, we often opt for the EASIER option because we are trying to get to the next thing. The trick here is to make this work in our favour rather than against us, by making it as easy as possible to make nourishing, mindful, intentional choices. This involves making them easier to see and access, because the more obvious the better!

This is how I get this to happen in our house. I keep a box of chopped-up vegetables at the front of our fridge, so it is the first thing we all see and the easiest thing to access when anyone opens the fridge. Put a damp piece of paper towel on the top and bottom of the veges to stop them drying out. This veg box works like a dream. I have often watched my husband walk into the kitchen looking for something to eat; left to his own devices he would stand in front of the pantry munching on crackers or chocolate or be taking the block of cheese out of the fridge and devouring big hunks. But instead, now he opens up the veg box and starts munching away! This gives him a minute or two to engage his brain and think about what he really wants to eat next, plus it gets him eating more veges, which is a win.

In the cooler months, I make a batch of soup on the weekend and put some in a pourable jug which sits in the door of the fridge, making it easy to access for lunch or as part of a mid-afternoon snack rather than picking at whatever is hanging around.

ACTION TIME! While it would be great if we all walked into the kitchen knowing exactly what we wanted to eat — which in time can come if you practise mindful eating — this is not always going to be the reality. So setting up your environment to be supportive of your goals can be really helpful.

- Want to eat more fruit? Put some out on the bench rather than hiding it all away in the fridge.
- Keen to have less coffee? Put herbal teas and decaf at the front of your cupboard so you see them first and they are easy to get.
- Looking to have more alcohol-free days? Have non-alcoholic drink options readily available and easy to see.
- Want your kids to make more nourishing snack choices? Make them easier to access (and put the other options out of reach).
- Keen to up your hydration? Fill up two drink bottles in the morning when you are making your breakfast — take one to work and work through the other one when you get home.

You can see where I am going here. This is all about making it EASIER and more obvious to make choices that support your wellbeing. It means creating helpful triggers for healthier habit loops. Chapter 9 has some extra tips on making new habits easier to adopt (see page 207), so there is more coming on this one to help you!

Forward thinking

Despite the many, many downsides of 'diets' and 'diet plans', there are understandable reasons why they are so popular. Firstly, they give you focus and make it easy to go shopping because you know what to buy. The structure that diets and plans offer helps, critically, with decision fatigue. And following a 'diet' alongside other people can give you a sense of identity if you find a group of people who eat the same way you do.

However, as you and I both know, restrictive diets and diet plans don't work and can really mess up your eating . . . So how do we take the best bits and leave the damaging bits behind?

Enter forward thinking! Essentially, this embraces the fundamental reason why 'diets' are attractive . . . they make it easier to make decisions about what to eat. This is where planning comes in.

Getting planning to become a habit was the entire reason I created my first wellbeing planner called 'It's a Beautiful Day', and other such tools that you can find on my website. They help you look at your week, at what is coming up that might influence your eating (be that meetings, social occasions or travel), and make a rough plan about how you will manage things. It then encourages you to plan what you will make for dinners, lunches and any breakfasts. From there, you can sort your shopping list.

Of course, this requires an investment in time initially, and to make it a habit you need to do it every week. Within a month or so, however, you will find it much easier and making intentional decisions about food will be much simpler. Something that following a plan from someone else doesn't help you do. It does not engage you in the process. To rewire your brain, you HAVE to be part of the process so this becomes part of who you are.

Use food subscription boxes if you need to make dinnertimes easier, or order your groceries online, and have some quick and easy go-to meals you can throw together on busy nights when the plan goes out the window — all these things help. But making the plan in the first place is the key to putting you back in the driving seat of your choices. Not just because it helps you have the right food in the house, but more because it helps you see the bumps in the road, the things that might trigger unhelpful eating habits, before they hit.

Accountability is important, too. Call your best friend, give them a copy of this book and get them on board with this process as well! Or get a group of you working on this together, sharing recipes, ideas and how you are doing. Follow me on social media, too, as I will be able to support you through this process with what I share.

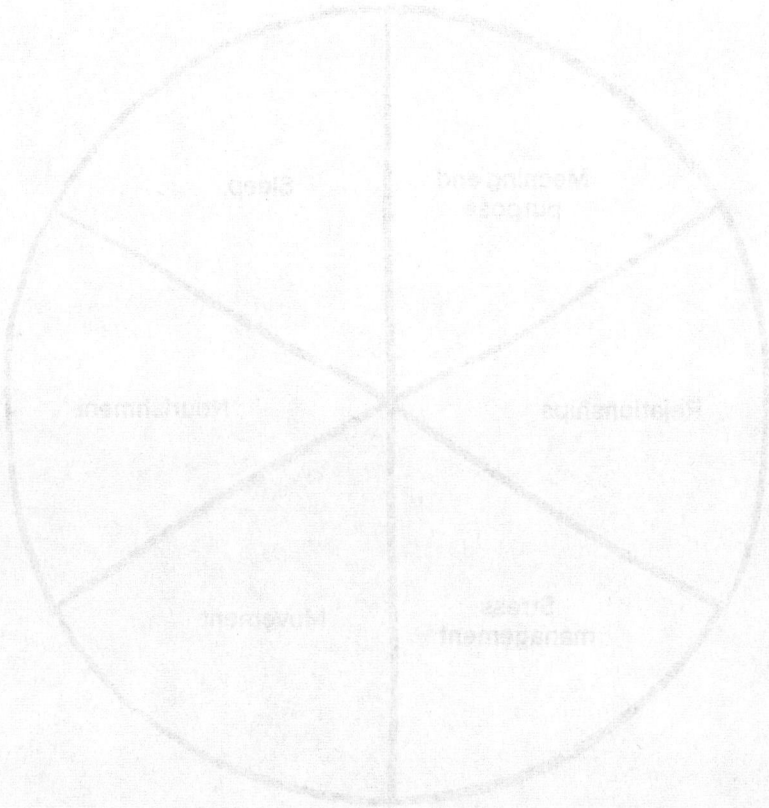

Chapter 9
Movement

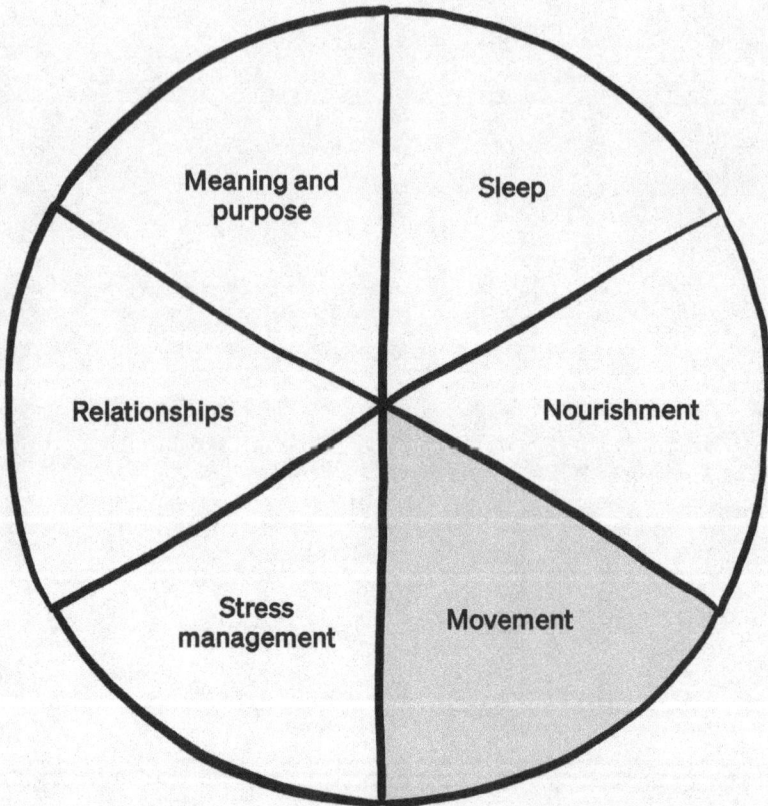

Moving your body has a profound effect on your physical and mental wellbeing. Way, way back in our evolutionary history, being highly physically active was a normal part of everyday life. It is estimated that in the few remaining hunter-gatherer tribes that still exist today, men take around 18,500 steps a day on average and women at least 13,000. This isn't just in the form of bog-standard walking, either; it includes fast-paced moments which really pump up the heart rate, as well as natural strength training in the form of lifting and carrying things that are required for day-to-day survival.

Currently, government guidelines recommend we do five hours of moderate physical activity or two and a half hours of vigorous physical activity each week. And, if you can, a bit more can be better. It is also recommended that we do some muscle-strengthening activities on at least two days each week. Regular muscle strengthening and weight-bearing activities help reduce the risk of developing metabolic syndrome, osteoporosis and osteoarthritis and of having falls and fractures. Important stuff! Unfortunately, though, 55% of adults in New Zealand are not reaching this recommendation, which is one reason why so many people are struggling with their health and wellbeing here. This is a trend that is common across much of the Western world.

Movement improves your mood, helps you sleep better, improves your cognitive function, helps you manage stress, and can enhance your immune function, improve your longevity and reduce your risk of chronic diseases like type 2 diabetes and some cancers. It also helps improve your insulin sensitivity, which is good news for all of us but particularly those of us with PCOS (polycystic ovary syndrome) or who are going through perimenopause/menopause.

If you are doing some strength training, this will also help increase your muscle mass — which is the best thing you can do to boost your metabolic rate. A higher metabolic rate means that your body is able to be more efficient and burns more calories even at rest, which is a really helpful thing for a lot of people.

On top of all this, movement can be an opportunity to socially interact with other people, which is really good for your wellbeing as well as providing opportunities for personal growth and achieving a sense of accomplishment that can lead to improved self-confidence and self-esteem.

Having struggled with depression on and off since I was 19, I have come to realise that movement is an absolute priority for me to keep myself afloat. Within a week of not exercising, whether on or off medication, I can go into some very dark spaces in my mind. As a result, exercise has become non-negotiable for me. Wherever I am, whatever I am doing, moving my body has to be part of my daily routine.

Making movement happen

When it comes to movement, it is one thing to understand the benefits but quite another to make it happen! That is the hardest part, right? Physical activity is often something we tell ourselves we will do when everything else is done, or we'll start next week, after the school holidays, or as soon as this busy patch at work passes. But there will always be a reason why it is too hard to get started or keep it going.

If you are currently in a good routine, wicked! Keep it up. You will still find what is coming up helpful, so keep reading.

If you are in need of a boost of motivation to get into a good groove of being more active, then help is here.

Again, it's about creating realistic goals and habits that stick.

Creating helpful habits

The following are the key elements in making healthy habits happen. As well as creating helpful habits around movement, these principles can be used to set up new habits of any sort — be it eating more veges, drinking more water, getting more sleep, or creating a mindfulness practice routine.

SET UP THE HABIT LOOP

There's a famous quote by Olympic runner Jim Ryun: 'Motivation is what gets you started; habit is what keeps you going.' I feel this sums up things pretty well. To make movement part of your everyday life it needs to become a habit, something that happens without you having to think much about it or rely on willpower to get on with it. You essentially have to set up a new habit loop. Below is a reminder of what that looks like.

To set up a habit loop, you first need to create a solid plan. This involves setting up triggers to kick off the loop, and making it as easy as possible for the movement (behaviour) to happen. If at first the reward of the movement isn't strong enough in itself, consider whether you need an additional reward to make it more appealing as you work to set up the habit.

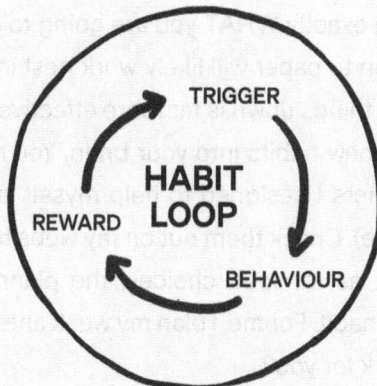

Then it is practise, practise, practise until this habit becomes integrated into your life. The same applies for any other new healthy habit you want to build, from eating better to making mindfulness part of your daily life.

MAKE THE PLAN

Planning is a form of pre-commitment, and is an essential part of making your healthy habits come to life and become subconsciously ingrained. Planning requires you to consciously take action by writing things down, and as you repeat this process over and over it will become easier and easier for your new habit to become your 'new normal'.

As with food choices, another advantage of planning is that it allows you to see the bumps in the road that might lead you off-course *before* you hit them. If, for example, you plan to go for a long walk four times a week and do three weights sessions at home, you must know whether the other commitments you have in the week might hinder this plan. If you are able to identify challenges before they arise, you can work around them. So, say you have two evening events coming up that are at the same time you would normally go for a walk. You can plan to do your walks at other times or fit in two shorter walks if needed.

I highly recommend getting yourself a weekly planner where you can write down exactly WHAT you are going to do, WHEN and WHERE. Putting pen to paper will likely work best initially — in my experience, writing things down is far more effective than anything else at embedding new habits into your brain. You may have seen the wellbeing planners I designed to help myself and others with this (and much more). Check them out on my website.

Remember, just as for food choices, the planning itself also needs to become a habit. For me, I plan my week ahead on a Sunday night. What will work for you?

BE SPECIFIC AND REALISTIC

When it comes to creating any new healthy habit, it's helpful from the get-go to be as **specific** as possible about what the new habit is going to be. So rather than just saying that your new habit will be to 'do more exercise', it could be 'do four walks a week'. The same applies when you are building a habit related to any part of the Wheel of Wellbeing, such as nourishment. Rather than saying you are going to 'eat better', break it down into what that means in terms of action steps, like 'eating five handfuls of vegetables a day' or 'packing nourishing snacks for work'.

As you work through the process of defining your new habit, be sure to consider whether what you are aiming for is **realistic**. It can be tempting to aim too high at the start when you are keen and motivated, but when you only walk three times a week when you told yourself you would go every day, you will feel like you have failed. Focus on starting small with a strong habit loop to kickstart things, then build on the size of your goal over time. In this case, that might be starting with four walks a week.

Being realistic is super-relevant to habits involving movement, as it's easy to push yourself too hard, too soon and then get injured! If you haven't done much exercise for a couple of years, starting with an hour's walk or run every day is probably unrealistic. Twenty minutes might be a better place to start, then build it up as you go. Even five minutes would be better than nothing. Remember to add in a habit of stretching afterwards, too!

Essentially, you need to make sure that with any new healthy habit you commit to, the baseline is something that you *really* have time to do. Aim for a small change that you *know* you can make, and it will be easier to create your new habit. If it is something you really enjoy, that will also make it so much easier.

If you have previously been really fit, I know it can be a bit mind-boggling not to set a big goal and smash it . . . but unless you have the time and space to do that consistently in the life stage you are in right now, it will only lead to disappointment.

I experienced this after having both my children. From once being able to lift heavy weights and do more burpees with ease than I care to remember, I barely had the energy to walk to the letter box. I felt like if I wasn't doing my hard-core hour a day of exercise it wasn't worth doing any, but that mindset got me nowhere. Eventually, I came to accept that in this new season of my life I needed to downsize the expectations I put on myself — and then downsize them again. I landed on 10 minutes of weights in the morning and a 15-minute walk around the block with the pram in the afternoon, extending that if it felt right on the day. It worked. A new habit was formed which fitted in with my new timetable and commitments. It was 152 hours more exercise in a year than I would have done if I had done nothing.

'Aim for progress, not perfection.'
— Unknown source

TRIGGERS OR HABIT ANCHORS
Two incredibly strong triggers for your habits are **time** and **location**. If you reflect back on the unhelpful habits you are trying to reprogram around eating, you will no doubt notice that they often happen in the same place and at a similar time — for example, eating cookies

on the couch after the kids have gone to bed, feeling uncomfortable eating in front of other people, or having a fourth coffee in the afternoon at work in the staff kitchen. The anchor of the time or location, or both, triggers the behaviour.

You can flip this in reverse for the new healthy, helpful habits you are trying to work on. What time will these habits happen? And where will you be?

Let's start with the example of drinking more water. You have decided that a realistic goal is six glasses of water a day on top of the two cups of herbal tea you currently have.

Now let's get specific on TIME and LOCATION. When will you drink this water? And where will you be?

- You decide to have one glass in your kitchen at home after you wake up — approximately 6.30 a.m.
- You take a 1 litre bottle of water (equivalent to four glasses) to work and drink it at your desk throughout the day.
- You then have a glass of water as soon as you get home from work (6.15 p.m.), in the kitchen before doing anything else.

When it comes to exercise, you might find it much easier to do something consistently every day at the same time than a couple of times a week. A few years ago, I set a goal of doing weights in my spare room at 6 a.m. three days a week, on Monday, Wednesday and Friday, and then let myself sleep longer on the other two weekdays. This didn't work out well. If I was too tired on Monday, I just told myself I would do it on Tuesday — which sometimes I did and some-times I didn't. This inconsistency just kept on going because I wasn't in the habit of getting up at the same time every day.

When I cottoned on to what was happening, I changed my plan. I would get up every day at the same time, so that the trigger was consistent, and do weights Monday, Wednesday and Friday, and stretching or yoga on the other two days. If I had heaps of work on, I sometimes used these two additional early mornings to smash through that if needed. The new plan worked out way better because it was more consistent. I ended up sleeping better overall and found it much easier to wake up at the same time each day.

With exercise, sometimes the location is obvious — like going to the gym or doing yoga in your living room — but if you do something like biking or walking without a plan of where you are going to go beforehand, it can be all too easy to talk yourself out of going at all. Plan your routes in advance and make that planning a habit, too.

Having reminders can also act as additional prompts to start your habit loop. I have alarms on my phone that remind me to do my workouts, meditate before bed and drink water. My kids have 'drink water' written in permanent marker inside their lunchboxes. I also have recurring appointments in my calendar for walks when my kids are at after-school activities. Be it alarms, sticky notes or big signs on your fridge, try using additional prompts or reminders to assist as extra triggers.

The more you repeat a habit, the more ingrained it becomes. It is not about taking 21 days to form a new habit, as people often say — it's about how many times you repeat that habit. Repeat it more often and it will be ingrained more quickly. Repeat it less often and it will take longer.

When a positive habit has become ingrained, you also have the advantage of cravings pushing you to do the behaviour, but this time with a good outcome! If you get into the routine of getting up earlier every morning to move your body, then as long as you are getting enough sleep you won't have to use much willpower to get you out of bed; it will have become your new normal. This is the secret of people who look like they are 'naturally healthy': they often have really good habits.

Keeping it going

Here are some useful tips and tricks to help you make your new habits stick:

Stack it

One way to make it more likely that you do a new habit is to 'stack it' on top of another habit. I need to take medication every morning, for example, so I have stacked this habit with brushing my teeth. My meds live in the bathroom next to my toothbrush; I see them when I go to brush my teeth and it reminds me to take them.

If you want to move your body more, you could stack this by doing a 15-minute power-walk every morning after dropping your kids at school or before heading into work, or after shutting down your laptop at the end of the day, or after you have finished washing up the dinner dishes — or before the dishes if that process might stop you from wanting to go for the walk.

Make it easy

Part of making any habit *actually* happen is making the behaviour as easy as possible to do, thus removing as many of the barriers as possible. Here are a few examples of how to make that happen:

- Committed to doing yoga in the morning? Lay your mat out in the living room before you go to bed.
- Going to the gym after work? Pack your gym bag the night before and leave it with your work bag so it is easy to grab in the morning. Consider leaving some spare gym clothes at work, too, in case you ever forget your gym bag, to make it easier for you to keep up this habit!

- Building the habit of early-morning runs? Get your exercise clothes and trainers ready the night before and put them by your bed as a visual prompt for you in the morning.
- As I mentioned earlier, it is also much easier to move your body when you enjoy what you are doing. You don't have to run, go to the gym or do yoga if that is not your thing! There are endless other ways to enjoy moving your body, from dancing to martial arts. Find what works for *you*.

'Make it so easy you can't say no.'

— Leo Barbuta, creator of Zen Habits

The little things count, too

As well as planning regular movement activities like walking, running, going to the gym, biking or swimming, it is super-important to consider ways to increase the amount of incidental activity you do in a day. Small changes that happen every day can really add up, so don't underestimate the impact these tweaks can make over time.

AT WORK

- Walk up the stairs instead of taking the lift.
- Cycle or walk to work instead of driving.
- Get off the train or bus a few stops earlier, or park further away, and walk to work from there. Reverse the process on the way home.
- Organise a regular exercise session at work and encourage everyone to get involved.
- Leave the office during your lunch break and go for a 10–15-minute walk.
- Walk around the office during calls if you can.
- Try the new coffee place a few blocks over, instead of the one in your building.
- Walk over to talk with a colleague instead of sending an email.
- Keep a pair of comfortable walking shoes at work — this gives you one less excuse not to exercise.
- Use a fitness tracker — most phones these days have one that will track the number of steps you do per day. Try to beat your daily target and increase your goal over time.
- Take 'active breaks' throughout the day, such as doing some desk exercises or taking the long route to the toilets.
- See if there is an option to get a stand-up desk.

AT HOME

- Go for a short walk before breakfast or after dinner.
- Be active while watching TV — for example, ride an exercise bike or walk on a treadmill.
- Perform squats or calf raises while waiting for the kettle to boil or for the microwave timer to count down.

- If you don't have a dog, take someone else's dog for a walk.
- Start 'Active Ads' — during TV commercials, do something active like squats, walking to the bedroom and back, or some exercises to strengthen your core.
- Challenge yourself to do the washing, vacuuming or mopping a bit quicker, to work up a sweat.
- Take smaller loads of washing up/down the stairs (or from room to room) rather than doing it in one large go.
- Do the housework instead of hiring someone to help.
- Do some gardening or mow the lawn.

TO BREAK UP LONG PERIODS OF SITTING

- Stand up to stretch often — for at least a few minutes each hour. Do this every time the ads come on TV.
- Stand while travelling on buses, trains and ferries.
- Limit TV, computer and other electronic device use when you are at home. Go for a walk instead.
- Stand up while texting or talking on the phone.

TO MAKE YOUR LEISURE TIME MORE ACTIVE

- Park further away from the shopping centre, cinema or sports ground and walk the extra distance.
- While at the shops, add in an extra lap of the centre.
- If you have kids who are playing, get involved in the game. Or walk around the field while you're watching them.
- Walk at golf instead of using a buggy.
- Walk along the beach before or after you swim.
- Organise active family outings — kick or throw a ball at the park, go for a bush walk, hire push-bikes for the afternoon, or head down to the local pool for a swim.

- Keep a soccer ball, skipping rope or Frisbee in the car.
- Walk to your local restaurant/shops/cafe instead of driving.
- Meet friends for a takeaway coffee, then catch up and chat while walking.

Financial commitment

For some habits it can be helpful to take your commitment to your goals a step further by financially investing in what you aim to do. Allocating money to your new desired habit may make it more likely to happen. For example, you might pre-pay for exercise classes before work. This might help motivate you to get out of bed in the morning to avoid that horrible feeling of $20 being wasted by you staying under the covers.

This also works for setting up helpful habits around food choices. Signing up to a veg subscription box that turns up every week might inspire some creative cooking action — and investing the money upfront hopefully means that the veges won't get wasted.

Set a future goal

In some cases, you can boost your commitment to a new habit by having a goal to work towards. This might be booking a Great Walk hike that you have to pay for in advance, to encourage you to get fit enough to do it; or it could be a bike race, or a holiday with an activity that you really want to do like diving or swimming, or one where you want to have plenty of energy so you can really enjoy things when you get there!

This year, to support my new habit of cycling, I committed to two long bike rides with friends who I wouldn't want to let down without good reason. We booked in specific dates and times, and I even booked accommodation in advance as a form of pre-commitment and financial investment to my goal. I also booked in a hike with a friend which was beyond my current level of fitness but a realistic goal in the time frame I have. This means that on days when it is raining or I am not in the mood, I still get myself up because I don't want to let my friends down. I also know that the hike and the rides will be so much easier if I am fitter, and that motivates me to get my trainers on and get out the door.

Be mindful of the goals you choose, though — don't set a goal that involves you needing to track your weight or size! Instead, select something that is more constructive. This applies to all new habits, whether they're related to food, drink or exercise.

Having someone to help you be accountable for your new habits is also useful. This could be a friend, family member or colleague who is keen to work on the same habits as you, or a health professional who can help by holding you accountable while you are working on making your new habit loop second nature.

I also find visual motivation to be helpful. I love quotes that remind me of what I am working towards; I have these as my phone background, on my fridge and in frames on my office wall by my desk. You might also like to create a vision board, too, something I do quite often — collecting pictures that inspire and motivate you can be helpful.

Rewards to support a new habit

Some healthy habits are naturally rewarding, like the high you get after a workout or how good you feel after eating a nutrition-packed lunch, but sometimes, especially at first, the kick isn't enough to motivate you to continue to complete the loop.

I personally really like the satisfaction of ticking things off a list, so I use my magnetic habit tracker (you can get it on my website).

It's a super-easy, affordable way to feel like I am getting a reward. Some people find that putting a marble or something similar in a jar every time they do their habit works for them — when the jar is full, they buy something for themselves, or organise a memorable experience they wouldn't normally do, or donate some money to a charity close to their heart. If you try this, choose something that you know is motivating for you and will make you happy.

You could also set up a 'healthy habit bank account'. When you complete a healthy habit you have committed to, you transfer money into that account. It could be 20 cents, $1 or $5 — whatever works and feels realistic and achievable for you. You can put any money you would otherwise have spent on an unhelpful habit into this bank account, too! Say you were bored, but instead of eating a doughnut you went for a 15-minute walk instead; put $3.50 in your account. If you went for a run instead of sitting on the couch browsing social media, pop $2 through.

It is really important to do these little money transfers as soon as practical after you have completed the healthy habit. If you can't or don't want to set up a real bank account, keep track on your phone or a note pad as soon as you have made the healthier choice, then tally it up at the end of the month!

Create a supportive environment

It can be extremely useful to create a supportive environment around you that helps make your new healthy habits feel normal and more achievable. Part of this might be having accountability partners, as mentioned earlier, but another layer is considering how you can be more in touch with people who are already doing the behaviours you are working to include more often in your life.

First things first: make sure you clean up your social media feed and unfollow all those people who are reinforcing diet culture messages, or have far more time to exercise than you do, or who often make you feel like you are failing because you aren't able to do what they do.

Next, look for inspiring and motivating people whose words *and* actions align with your vision of a more balanced, self-compassionate version of you. People who fit movement into a life that feels more like yours, who share tips and advice that feels **practical and realistic** for you. If you need any ideas, look through the list of people I follow.

Next, seek to spend more time with people who have lives that align with your goals and new habits. If you are wanting to walk more, join a hiking club or walking group, or connect with friends who you know are equally committed to setting up regular dates to get moving. If you want to eat better, connect with people who are interested in home cooking, growing their own veges or making quick-and-easy nutritious meals. Find people whose values and vision align with yours.

'Act as if you were already the person you most want to be.'

— motivational speaker Brian Tracy

Believe in yourself

As I said in Chapter 1 and discussed in the context of self-sabotage in Chapter 5, your beliefs create your reality. **You need to *believe* that you can make positive changes in your life to make it possible for them to happen.** This means that despite what has happened in your life so far, it is time to challenge the story you keep telling yourself.

You *can* become fitter, you *can* become strong, you *can* feel better about yourself. But first you must believe that this is possible.

As one of my all-time favourite quotes goes: 'Believe you can, and you are halfway there.' That's from former US president Theodore Roosevelt.

———

One final note. Like much of the rest of my life, and no doubt yours, too, my movement habits go through ups and downs, twists and turns. When the seasons change, routines change as well. You will need to check in regularly to see how things are going with your commitment to movement — and to see what changes you need to make, because, for most people, things will change over time.

Once again, **don't be hard on yourself** if you were in a good routine and then things didn't stay that way. There is always a chance to regroup and start again.

Chapter 10
Stress management

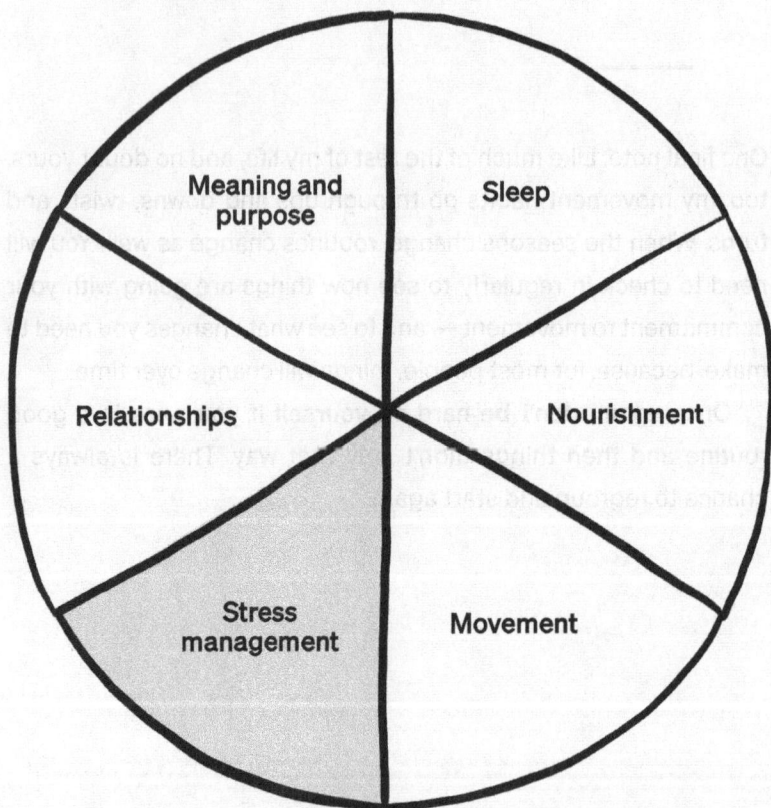

Meaning and purpose

Sleep

Relationships

Nourishment

Stress management

Movement

There is a lot of talk about stress these days, and with the pressures of our busy modern world it really is no surprise! But what actually *is* stress? And how can you manage things better so stress doesn't take over your life?

First up, **stress isn't inherently bad, and there is a very good reason why we have an inbuilt stress response.** In days gone by when life was a lot simpler, stress came in the form of large wild animals wanting to eat us, or a neighbouring tribe wanting to take over our land. In these circumstances, our bodies needed to take action — and fast — so we could either run for our lives or stand up and fight in order to survive.

Stress typically activates your body's sympathetic nervous system, more commonly known as the system that activates your 'fight or flight' response. This makes your heart rate increase, your adrenaline spike, your eyes be more focused, and your body rustle up all available resources so you are ready to take on the danger approaching!

Provided you escaped from the animal or survived the battle, your body would then return to a more relaxed, calm state, and the parasympathetic part of your nervous system would be activated. This is known more commonly as the 'rest and digest' state, and is where your body likes to be much of the time.

However, with its traffic jams, financial stresses, deadlines, relationship challenges, crammed inboxes, juggling of a million kids' activities, endless 'pinging' sounds of notifications, weather events and suchlike, our modern world means that our sympathetic nervous system is activated far more often than is healthy. Sometimes, it gets almost permanently switched on, which can lead to feelings of overwhelm, chronic stress and, at worst, a nervous system breakdown.

This is something I know about all too well. On 23 December 2020, amid a very stressful situation, I collapsed on the floor.

Unable to get up, I lay there for what seemed like an eternity before managing to crawl to my bed — and there I stayed. I had no idea what had happened or why I fell to the floor; I only knew that there was definitely something seriously wrong. My memory was intermittent, I couldn't talk properly, and I was unable to make sense of sounds. I waited it out a few days, attempted to be a functioning human on Christmas Day with my family, but ended up back in bed, terrified of what was happening.

On the 28th, as I wasn't feeling any better, I decided to go to the doctor. I sat there trying to explain what had happened, but clearly I wasn't making much sense; my thoughts and conversation were all over the place. After a thorough examination and lengthy questioning, my doctor suggested the most likely explanation was a brain tumour and I was urgently referred for a CT scan and an MRI. The days between my doctor's appointment and the scans actually being done felt like the longest I have ever experienced in my life. And the hour I was in the MRI machine is something I will never, ever forget — not just the loud sounds and the sense of claustrophobia, but also lying there on my own contemplating my life and wondering what might happen if it was to be the worst news. *How will I tell the kids I might die?*

Luckily, there was no tumour to be found; but there was also no explanation for my collapse. I was put on a waiting list to see a neurologist, which, due to Covid-related delays, was a long one. When I finally saw the neurologist and spent 90 minutes being examined, he concluded that I'd essentially had a nervous system collapse — a bit like a heart attack, but affecting my brain instead of my heart. The neurologist thought that because I had a virus at the time of the 'attack', a stressful situation on top of my already frazzled nervous system was enough to push me over the edge.

The treatment? He said it would be 3–5 years minimum of managing myself as if I had experienced a severe concussion. I was not to underestimate how long it would take to heal and how hard it would be. He insisted that I was not to do high-intensity exercise, that I would need to sleep as much as possible, take rests in the day, limit screen time, limit exposure to sounds and bright lights, and it would be highly likely I would need to do this for a long time.

When I walked out of the consultation room after hearing all this, I thought to myself, *this doctor doesn't know me and how motivated I am — I will be back to my old self in no time.*

How wrong I was.

I didn't go into a restaurant or cafe for about 18 months because of the effect the light and the noise had on me. The first time I did, my friend Kavita kindly agreed to come with me at 5 p.m. to test things out and see if I could do it. I was forced to leave as soon as the food arrived at the table because I felt like I was about to collapse again with all the sounds in the room. I cried myself to sleep that night.

Supermarkets were an absolute nightmare because of the noise and bright lights, so online shopping became my go-to. If I did have to go into a store, I needed ear plugs or noise-cancelling headphones just to get through the door. And then I also needed to spend the next few days at home with as little noise around me as possible. I ended up wearing ear plugs all day long just so I could manage the noise of the kids and things as minor as the kettle boiling or the extractor fan being on.

Things weren't any easier when it came to work, either. I couldn't do any TV, radio or speaking work properly for about a year. If I did do any high-energy-output work, I would end up in bed for days afterwards. Initially I had to limit my screen use to about 30 minutes, and then had to close my eyes and block out all sound for at least 20 minutes to be able to get back to it. If I didn't, my speech would go and I would be literally unable to function. Nine hours of sleep a night became a non-negotiable bare minimum, with ten or more being better, and I couldn't drink any alcohol or caffeine at all.

When you have children, you feel like you lose yourself in a way because your life changes so much so quickly, but this breakdown was even harder than that transition. I totally lost myself and my confidence. The things I loved doing at work were no longer possible; I couldn't listen to the music I loved or go out other than on my own, somewhere very quiet. I looked normal on the outside, but on the inside I felt broken, lost and scared. I didn't know how long life would be like this or if I would ever be myself again.

For many years leading up to the day I collapsed, in many ways I was dealing with a lot of stress in my personal life, much of which was unavoidable and mostly out of my control. I was getting help with therapy, and I was exercising to help relieve anxiety. Admittedly, on reflection I was also working more than was healthy given the other commitments in my life, because work makes me feel good and was something in my life I *could* control. I had been, for the most part, coping and working through things in a positive way. But then Covid times hit. My husband still needed to work full-time, nine to five, so (given that my work is more flexible) I ended up getting up at 4.30 a.m. and working until nine, then looking after the kids all day, then working from 5 p.m. until ten and sometimes much later. I then also worked all weekend. Like everyone else, I was trying to figure out how to keep things going. How to restructure my own business as well as keep Mission Nutrition and my team there afloat so we could all somehow still make enough money to pay the rent or mortgage and put food on the table.

For a while, it seemed to be working. I was getting everything done and having some fun adventures with the kids during the daytime, exploring nature and filming cool content, recipes and lockdown ideas for my social media. However, the added stress on top of the previous years of challenges eventually took its toll. The high-intensity exercise I had been doing for years because it served me well was now pushing my body too far given the stress and sleep deprivation I was experiencing. The work that once gave me so much joy was becoming so pressured that I felt, as did many others, like I was drowning. I was also worried about my family overseas: not knowing whether I would see my parents in the UK again was dreadful. It is no wonder that I, like so many others, had a nervous system collapse.

———

There are many things I have learnt about myself from this experience, but the biggest lesson of all has been that no matter what, you can't cheat your body. As renowned psychiatrist and trauma expert Dr Bessel van der Kolk puts it: 'Your body keeps the score.' When things are going on inside you, they will always make their presence known on the outside — be this in the subconscious choices you make or the health issues that emerge.

Since my collapse, I have studied stress and its impact on the body and mind with great interest. At the time, while I was doing the basics right — like eating well, trying to sleep well and keeping active — there were all sorts of things I was missing when it came to managing stress and avoiding overwhelm. It is those tools and techniques that I want to share with you so that, hopefully, you never have to go through what I did by pushing things too far for too long.

The World Health Organization says: 'Stress can be defined as a state of worry or mental tension caused by a difficult situation. Stress is a natural human response that prompts us to address challenges and threats in our lives. Everyone experiences stress to some degree. The way we respond to stress, however, makes a big difference to our overall well-being.'

That last part is key. **Stress is sometimes unavoidable, but there are ways to manage it with the right support and approach.**

Causes of stress — what's in your control and what's not

There are some things in our lives that we can control, and others that we can't. We can't control whether or not someone we know is diagnosed with a terminal illness. We can't control the weather, the financial position of the country we live in or, often, how much we get paid to do what we do.

We can't always know how other people feel about us, how our bosses will act, how other people will talk or respond to us, and nor can we change who other people are at their core. As much as we would like to sometimes!

There are, however, some things that add to our stress which we can control.

We can control our boundaries and what we give our energy to, including the additional things we commit to outside of what is required to keep the basics of life in order. I appreciate that this is easier said than done sometimes, especially if you find it hard to say no, because you don't like letting people down or you are a people-pleaser. But **you matter, too**, and it is important to remember that you can't be everything to everybody. When you don't look after yourself, you can't be the best for anyone, including yourself. If you end up burning yourself out as a result of over-committing, no one wins. If you are someone who over-commits, you will probably need to look at the beliefs that lie underneath (we will look at this in Chapter 11; see page 253).

We can also control the goals we chase and how much that results in us pushing ourselves. Having dreams and working towards a goal can be super-healthy, but we can fall into the trap of always wanting more, pushing more and doing more, which often doesn't work out so well. If this is you, then it's time to ponder on that one.

Another thing we can look to control, or at least manage, is the people we choose to spend time with. Where we can't do that, we can at least choose how we react to people we are unable to distance ourselves from.

Lastly, we can control our thoughts, actions, attitude and how we speak to ourselves. These are perhaps the most important things to control and I will be covering this in Chapter 11 (see page 266). Often it is not the situation that is stressful in itself, but more how we are interpreting the situation in our heads based on the internal dialogue that goes on around it.

TIME TO REFLECT: Think about the things in your life that you feel cause you to be stressed. What is in your control that you might be able to take action on?

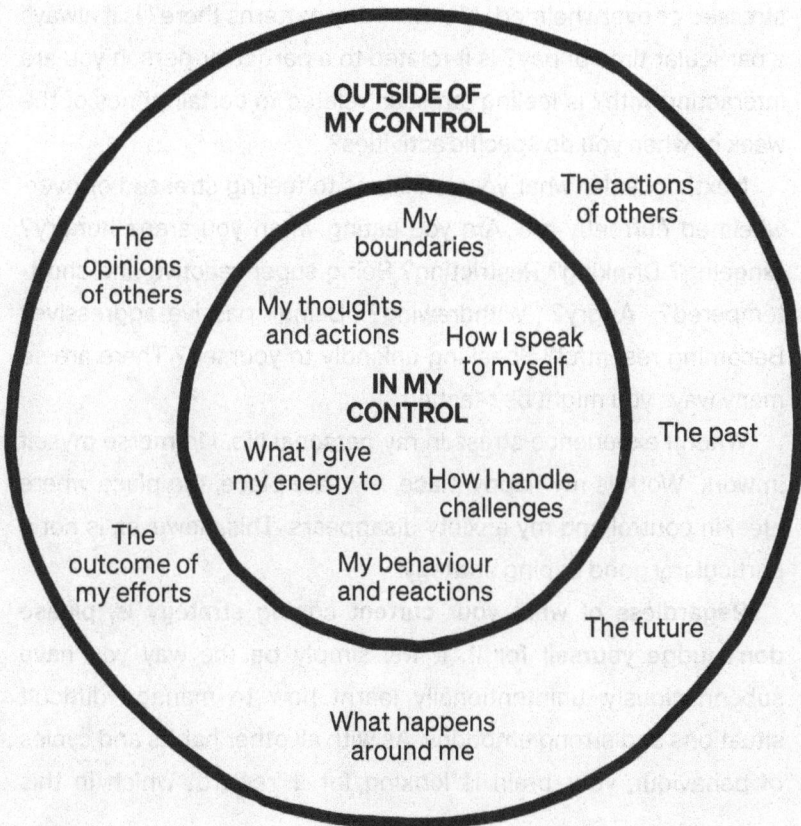

OUTSIDE OF
MY CONTROL

The actions
of others

My
boundaries

The
opinions
of others

My thoughts
and actions

How I speak
to myself

IN MY
CONTROL

The past

What I give
my energy to

How I handle
challenges

My behaviour
and reactions

The future

The
outcome of
my efforts

What happens
around me

Simple strategies to manage stress

Notice it and name it

In the same way that you need to become aware of your eating habits in order to reprogram them, you also need to become aware of what is contributing to how stressed and overwhelmed you are feeling. You need to know what the triggers are in order to be able to do something about it.

Getting things down on paper is a good first step. Try keeping a diary for a couple of weeks. In it, keep a record of the situations and circumstances that were present when you noticed feeling stressed or overwhelmed. Are there any patterns there? Is it always a particular time of day? Is it related to a particular person you are interacting with? Is feeling stressed related to certain times of the week or when you do specific activities?

Next, consider what your reactions to feeling stressed or over-whelmed currently are. Are you eating when you aren't hungry? Bingeing? Drinking? Restricting? Being super-reactive and short-tempered? Angry? Withdrawing? Being passive-aggressive? Becoming resentful? Speaking unkindly to yourself? There are so many ways you might be reacting.

When I experience stress in my personal life, I immerse myself in work. Work is my happy place, my safe place, the place where I feel in control and my anxiety disappears. This, however, is not a particularly good coping strategy.

Regardless of what your current coping strategy is, please don't judge yourself for it. It will simply be the way you have subconsciously, unintentionally learnt how to manage difficult situations and strong emotions. As with all other habits and cycles of behaviour, your brain is looking for a 'reward', which in this case will likely be having those feelings of stress and overwhelm dissipate, even if only very temporarily.

It can be really helpful to become more aware of your stress triggers and how you are reacting to them. This is, once again, done through the practice of mindfulness. As defined by the world-renowned expert in this area, Professor Jon Kabat-Zinn, mindfulness is 'awareness that arises through paying attention, on purpose, in the present moment, non-judgmentally'. Mindfulness can influence all aspects of our wellbeing, including our ability to manage stress.

Practising mindfulness can help you increase the gap between a trigger and your reaction, as we discussed on page 121. It is in this gap that you can change everything. This is possible when you become aware of the trigger (stimulus) before automatically reacting or cracking into your default response.

One very powerful quote that has completely changed my life is often attributed to the neurologist, psychologist and Holocaust survivor Viktor Frankl: 'Between stimulus and response there is a space. In that space is our power to choose our response. In our response lies our growth and our freedom.' While the origin of this quote is unclear, its message is powerful. (As a side note, if you haven't read any of Frankl's books, then Man's Search for Meaning is a must.)

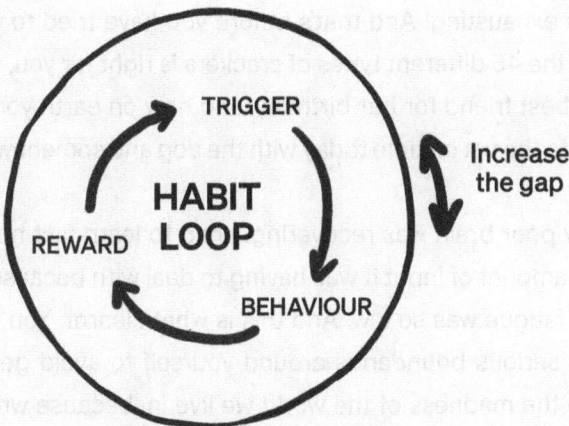

TRIGGER

HABIT LOOP

REWARD

BEHAVIOUR

Increase the gap

I encourage you to revisit Chapter 5 to recap on the process of reprogramming unhelpful eating behaviours, as reprogramming your stress responses can be approached in a similar way. Essentially, you are firstly looking to reduce the impact of the things that are triggering you to feel stressed, then secondly coming up with new responses to deal with feelings of stress when they do arise.

Below are some ideas that can help with both these things. There are also helpful ideas in the section on emotion regulation in Chapter 5 (see page 113).

Manage your data input

One thing I learnt from my nervous system collapse was just how bombarded our brains are with information all the time, and how many decisions we have to make minute by minute every day. It is not surprising that so many of us experience decision fatigue — which is finding it hard to make decisions when there is so much to think about, and in some cases far too many choices.

With phones at our fingertips, what feels like at least ten different messaging apps, endless appointments to keep up with to make sure that everything from your eyes to your teeth to your bowels are in order, it is exhausting! And that's before you have tried to work out which of the 45 different types of crackers is right for you, what to buy your best friend for her birthday, and how on earth you are going to get to the vet on time today with the dog and somehow pay for it, too.

When my poor brain was recovering, I had to learn fast how to manage the amount of input it was having to deal with because my capacity for fatigue was so low. And this is what I learnt. You have to set some serious boundaries around yourself to avoid getting sucked in to the madness of the world we live in, because while it has become 'normal' to get emails and messages every hour of the day and night, it is certainly *not* normal, nor helpful, when it comes to keeping ourselves mentally and physically well.

The first thing to do is be aware of how much input you are getting, by reviewing your screen time and how many times you pick up your phone a day. Go to your settings and look. On an Apple phone it is under 'Screen time'; on android it is currently under 'Settings' then 'Digital Wellbeing'. This stuff changes all the time, so do a search if you can't work out how to get the info for your phone. You might need to be prepared to be horrified.

It is estimated that, on average, an adult picks up their phone 144 times a day. I just checked mine as I am writing this: 72 times is my own average. It used to be lot worse a few years ago, but, wow, there is still a goal for me there. We have become conditioned to pick up these little blocks of metal in a way that is nothing more than terrifying. Yes, mobile phones are in part amazing and they have many benefits, but there is a difference between mindfully using one and being tethered to it as if your life depended on it.

If screen time isn't something that is a problem for you, this information could still be useful for your friends, partner, children, grandchildren, or to share with other people who seem tethered to their devices, so stay tuned.

If you think you can rely on willpower to use your phone less, you are very likely to be disappointed. In the same way that willpower can't be relied on to change the way we eat or drink in the long term, it sure as heck can't be relied on to change the way we interact with our phones. Many of the apps, particularly the social media ones, have been designed with the input of some of the best brains in neuroscience to make them highly addictive, meaning it is very difficult for you to stop interacting with them.

Addiction absolutely fascinates me, and it's another thing I have studied at length because it underpins so many of the challenges we face in many aspects of our modern world with its easy access to highly processed food, alcohol, drugs, pornography, gambling, gaming and, of course, computers and phones.

Anna Lembke, a leading American psychiatrist specialising in the area of addiction, defines addiction as 'the continued and compulsive use of a substance or behavior, despite harm to self and/or others'. When you become addicted to a behaviour or a substance, you have essentially created an incredibly strong habit loop that drives you towards it, as I talked about in Chapter 1 (see page 37). The cravings you experience with addictions are extremely powerful and can be experienced in your body as pain or a form of discomfort or agitation.

Have you ever felt uncomfortable when you haven't checked your phone or emails for a while, when you are used to interacting with them all the time? How about if you get a notification from Facebook or Instagram when you are in a meeting or out and about . . . it can feel like it's an itch you have to scratch. That is addiction in action.

Do you wake up every morning and mindlessly start scrolling before you even say good morning to the person lying next to you? Or have kids who are often watching you scrolling or typing while they are trying to engage with you? Sitting at dinner with friends and spending more time looking at your screens than looking each other in the eye? It might be normal in our modern world, but it is certainly not healthy and is not helping us live our best lives.

To help manage the input from your phone, here are a few things to try:

- Go to your settings and turn off all notifications for social media apps or those you find yourself checking often out of habit.
- In your settings, set time limits for the apps that you commonly use.
- While you are at it, get your phone to stop listening to your conversations and doing things like sending you dog-training recommendations after you chat to your friend about her new puppy. Again in settings, go to 'Privacy' and turn off your microphone. If you need your microphone on for some apps, like WhatsApp, you can selectively turn the microphone off on the other apps by tapping into each one's settings. Google how to do this if you need to. There are a lot of videos these days to help with things like this.
- Another thing I've personally found incredibly helpful is wearing a watch which is connected to my phone. It will ring if it is school, my husband, one of my team or anyone else I have marked as important, but it doesn't allow me to interact with any of my social media apps and means my phone can stay in a drawer, my bag or a pocket.
- Lastly, log out from your social media accounts during the day, and don't have your passwords autosaved. Also, don't have social media apps open on your work computer. You and I both know it is far too tempting if it is too easy.

BE INFORMED, NOT CONSUMED

The world is full of bad news, and it always has been, but now we can get to hear about it all the time, being updated minute by minute if we want to with all the graphic details of the ins and outs of whatever is going on. This can increase stress and makes us feel less in control. But becoming depressed and anxious about everyday life because the world feels so tragic doesn't help solve the problems around the world.

Yes, we do need to be across what is going on. We also need to fight for the causes that matter, stand up for the things we believe in and not accept that this is how the world should be. But we don't need to be so consumed by the moment-by-moment details of every police case around the world and of every war zone to the point where it completely consumes our own lives, compromises our wellbeing and paralyses us into inaction. This is something I experienced myself before taking a more mindful approach.

As the lovely psychologist Jacqui Maguire taught me during Covid, here is a message I pass on to you: 'Be informed, not consumed.'

Microbreaks

When my neurologist told me I needed to limit my screen time to 20–30 minutes at a time, and I might need to do this for quite a while, I thought it was totally ridiculous. I believed there was no way I could get my work done with that approach, so instead I tried to push through. Of course, it ended up being a disaster. I got crazy headaches that I couldn't shift, and after a couple of hours I couldn't think at all. I ended up in tears, frustrated with having the time to work but not being able to do anything other than stare at the wall.

Eventually I had to give in, and very reluctantly tried his approach of taking a brain break for 10–20 minutes every half-hour. At first, when I sat down on the couch with my eyes closed I was aware of the thoughts in my head saying over and over again, *what a waste of time this is*. Over time, however, I started to see that these small breaks made me much more productive in the 30 minutes that followed. The negative chatter in my brain got quieter, and in these short breaks I started to come up with all sorts of different ideas for business, articles, social media content as well as solutions to issues I was having with the kids or other problems I was trying to solve.

My 30 minutes of screen time started to push out to 45 minutes and then a full hour, but I still took my short breaks in between. Over time, I found that breaks of 5–10 minutes seemed to be enough to recharge me — *and* they were also really helping me get more out of my day, not less. I was becoming more productive, more efficient and more creative than ever before. Now, four years later, I do a full 90 minutes of focused work followed by a quick break and it is a habit I will never change. Even though I have more gaps in my day, I am more productive than ever.

How so? How can you be more efficient with less time?

Here's how. Your brain needs gaps to connect the dots between all the information that is thrown at it in the form of things you have seen, heard, read, said and so on. Historically, we would have had lots of time to do this — and even when I was growing up, without mobile phones in our hands all the time, there were always natural gaps in the day when your brain had nothing to do. Standing in a queue. Waiting at the bus stop. Walking down the street. Do you ever wonder why you have such good ideas when you are out walking without listening to anything, or in the shower, or lying in bed? It's because, *finally*, your brain has had a chance to connect those dots.

So often these days we fill gaps like these by looking at something, reading something or listening to something. Our poor brains need time to catch up on all the data they have had to take in *already* that day without us adding more in there! We have come to believe that to *be* more, we need to *do* more, but this just isn't true. When we give our body the time and space it needs to function as it is meant to, the results can be amazing. Some workplaces around the world are seeing the value of this and encouraging this practice for their staff, but it needs to be much more widely understood. I now truly believe in the phrases 'we need to work smarter not harder' and 'you can get more and be more by doing less'.

I appreciate that there are many work situations where a 5- to 10-minute sit-down with your eyes closed is completely impractical, but there are lots of things you can do to get small breaks for your brain to catch up during the day. Here are some:

AT WORK

- Leave your phone behind when you go to get a glass of water or make a cuppa, and notice your surroundings while you get your drink.
- When you get in a lift, leave your phone in your pocket.
- Heading to the loo? You don't need your phone!
- Going out to grab a coffee? Again, leave your phone on your desk or in your pocket, and just take your cash card.
- Have a device-free lunch break.
- If you are feeling tired, head outside and walk around the building, leaving your phone behind.
- Choose a quiet space and do ten press-ups, ten push-ups, squats or some simple stretches for 2–3 minutes to give your brain a break.

OUT AND ABOUT

- Drive without the radio on and just learn to be okay with simply focusing on driving. This helps you drive more safely, too!
- While waiting at the bus stop or train station, notice what's around you rather than scrolling on your phone. It might

feel uncomfortable at first, but that actually proves the point of how addictive technology can be.

- Allow yourself to just 'be' in a checkout queue without logging in to your emails or seeing what is happening on social media.

AT HOME

- Do washing up or folding the laundry mindfully, without the TV on or other data going into your brain at the same time.
- Cooking can be a great mindful activity. Shifting it from a chore to a mental health practice can make it more appealing.

Cold exposure

Cold-water therapy is becoming increasingly popular, whether in the form of ice baths, chilly dips in the ocean, or cold showers. The theory is that by exposing yourself to extremely cold water in a controlled environment, you can activate your body's stress response and train yourself to manage it by managing your breathing and thinking. Your body's automatic reaction will be to activate 'fight or flight' mode and your breathing will become short and shallow, but if you practise slow, deep breathing, you will be able to take control of your response and move back to a calmer state.

I have followed the cold-water trend with interest for many years now as the emerging research highlights some positive findings, including the potential to decrease inflammation in the body, positively impact your gut microbiome, improve your metabolic health and boost your mood and cognition. The WHO even added it to their recommendations in 2020 because of the benefits for mental and physical health.

Personally, I find it helps. I have yet to get into an ice bath or take a chilly ocean dip, but I do finish off my shower every morning with 1–2 minutes of cold water. I genuinely find that it helps me feel more alert, awake and focused. After doing this for over a year now, I also honestly feel that when I come across a stressful situation I am able to better control my breathing and my thinking than I did before.

So why not give it a try? Start with the cold-shower version and see if you notice any difference in how you feel, and whether you think this could be a helpful part of your daily routine. If you love it, you might end up being an ice-bath or chilly-dip convert!

A word of caution, however. If you consider yourself to be chronically stressed at the moment, this is *not* something I would recommend. Like high-intensity exercise, it may activate your stress response in a way that isn't helpful. Only try this when your stress is more under control. Also, if you have a heart condition, abnormal blood pressure, are over 50 or have any other medical concerns, or any concerns at all, it is best to check with your doctor before trying this, so ask them about it at your next checkup.

Research also suggests that as well as cold exposure, controlled heat exposure supports your wellbeing, too! So if you like saunas and steam rooms, and have access to them, this might be something to look into.

Breath work

At the end of my consultation with the neurologist, I had to do a breathing assessment — and it was clear from his face that he wasn't impressed. Apparently, when I was thinking, reading or focusing on something, I had the habit of holding my breath. My breathing was also generally shorter and shallower than it should be. Despite doing the odd yoga class with breathing lessons and knowing the ins and outs of the importance of breathing properly, I clearly wasn't doing it habitually myself. The neurologist was very clear that learning to breathe properly was an essential part of my recovery.

Prior to Covid, I had been really consistent with using the Calm app at night to do nightly meditations for 5–10 minutes, but when I started working really late this habit fell by the wayside. It was time to pick it back up again, and make it stick this time. After a couple of weeks of practising deep, slow belly breathing, also known as diaphragmatic breathing, in the evenings and also making it part of my microbreaks during the day, I did start to notice a difference regarding how anxious I was feeling and overall felt calmer.

Learning to breathe correctly is an incredibly powerful — and free — thing you can do to improve your wellbeing, and it can also help you manage feelings of stress and overwhelm. Short, shallow breathing is interpreted by your brain as danger and becomes part of the cycle that fires up your sympathetic nervous system's 'fight or flight' response. Slow, deep breathing, on the other hand, is the quickest and easiest way to activate your parasympathetic nervous system and the calming 'rest and digest' response. When your exhalation is longer than your inhalation this is also hugely advantageous.

How breathing works

Breathing is a complex process involving the lungs and the diaphragm, the ribs and the muscles of the abdomen and neck. During inhalation, the diaphragm contracts and moves downward, allowing air to flow into the lungs, while the ribcage expands to create space for the lungs to fill. During exhalation, the opposite happens. The diaphragm relaxes and moves upward, expelling the used air from the lungs.

Practising diaphragmatic breathing

You can do this standing, sitting or lying down:

- Close your eyes and put one hand on your chest and one on your belly.
- Now breathe in through your nose and notice which hand moves. Is it the hand on your chest? Or the hand on your belly?
- What you are aiming for is to breathe into your belly rather than your chest.
- There are all sorts of breathing combinations you can try. The one I like the most is breathing in for a count of 4, holding your breath for a count of 1, breathing out for a count of 8 and then holding for another count of 1, and repeating.

Making this your new automatic way of breathing, like any other habit, takes practice! If you are new to this practice, you might find lying down is best, with your eyes closed to help increase your awareness of what you are doing. You can also put something on your belly like a box of tissues, a wheat bag or pair of socks to see whether or not it is going up and down when you breathe.

Have a try and see how it makes you feel. If you can get into the habit of practising this every morning before you get up and every night before you go to bed, even just for 10–20 breaths, it can really help. It also means that when you are feeling stressed you have this tool in your kit, available to you at any time. At least a couple of times a week I do this during the day when I feel triggered by my kids' behaviour or get an email that makes me feel overwhelmed.

I also used the technique to help me manage my fear of flying. I used to fly in and out of Wellington every fortnight for a couple of years to film for what was TVNZ's *Good Morning* back in the day, and I always had a sleepless night leading up to it. I would literally be shaking the minute I sat down on the plane, and would have to warn the person sitting next to me that I might inadvertently grasp their hand or arm. Now, however, although I am still terrified, I can manage my body's stress response and get through it by closing my eyes and doing my 4, 1, 8, 1 breathing pattern. Given that I now live in Queenstown, whose airport isn't exactly the easiest or smoothest to get in and out of, it is a good job I have this problem (mostly) under control!

The power of movement

When I was a teenager, my mum used to wave my trainers under my nose and say 'Off you go' on the days when I was clearly struggling with how I was feeling. She knew that if I went outside and moved my feet, many of the things that were going round and round in my head and making me feel overwhelmed would be tamed in a spectacular way. Just by running up to our local woods, seeing the sea in the distance and getting some fresh air, life somehow seemed more manageable again when I returned home.

There really is nothing like the power of movement to change how you feel in a very short space of time. Moving your body helps you reduce your level of stress hormones, release feel-good endorphins, and get out of your own head for a while.

However, there are different approaches to movement that need to be taken depending on how much stress you are experiencing. I learnt this the hard way and want to save you from that.

- If you are in a phase of your life when you are mostly coping well, having the odd ups and downs, and feel your stress is mostly manageable using some of the tips in this book, then doing a wide variety of activities that get you moving regularly is a great goal. Aim for the recommended five hours of moderate exercise and a couple of strength-training sessions a week, and some high-intensity workouts if you have the time and are able to do them. Harder sessions and taking part in organised events might work well for you, too. Exercise helps build up your tolerance to stress, so this is a perfect time to get that into action.

- If you are currently feeling stressed a lot of the time, not sleeping that well and generally in quite a difficult phase, you need to reflect on how different types of movement make you feel. While it is good to keep aiming for the goal of five hours of moderate or two and a half hours of vigorous physical activity, you might find that high-intensity exercise actually makes you feel really exhausted and almost unwell afterwards. If this is you, then I suggest doing your workouts as speed walks, weights and adding some yoga into the mix rather than pushing through thinking that you just need to tough it out. Feeling tired and unwell might be the start of alarm bells warning that your body is really struggling and doing more could actually send you backwards.

This is advice I wished I had known when I was struggling in late 2020. I was finding it almost impossible to climb out of bed to get to the gym for my 5.30 a.m. class, sometimes crying on the way there because I was so tired. While I loved doing the class at the time, I felt terrible for most of the day afterwards even though I was eating properly and getting enough sleep.

I kept going, because in my mind was the message 'exercise helps stress' — but I now know that this is only true if you aren't on the edge of burnout, which I was. Pushing myself too far for too long definitely contributed to my nervous system collapse.

If you are currently experiencing chronic stress, really not sleeping well, feeling overwhelmed and constantly feeling like you are in fight or flight mode, please don't do what I did and try to run it off or go harder at the gym. This is the worst thing you can do if your body has been flooded with adrenaline far too often — it will lead to your sympathetic nervous system getting stuck in the 'on' position. As hard as it can be if you are a *go, go, go!* person, this is the time to choose walking over running, yoga and Pilates over CrossFit, and get your movement in more gentle ways.

This, as with the rest of the advice in this book, is about finding what works for *you*. **Listen to your body and learn to trust yourself again.**

Mini movement breaks

Alongside any walks, runs, Pilates classes, swims, biking, gym sessions or weight workouts that you do to prevent and manage stress, it can be really helpful to also include mini movement breaks throughout your day. These help keep your brain in optimal working order and prevent stress building up as you go through the day. How you do this will depend on whether you are in a workplace setting, out and about, or at home.

Nowadays I aim to work in 90-minute blocks and then do some kind of movement for at least 30 seconds to a minute, often as part of the 5- to 10-minute microbreaks I talked about on page 237. Sometimes this movement is running from my desk to the letter box, sometimes walking round my garden or running up and down my stairs. I also have dumbbells by my desk, so sometimes I do 20 squats, bicep curls or overhead pushes with them.

When I am waiting for the kettle to boil, I also often do a few squats in the kitchen or press-ups on my kitchen bench. Sometimes meetings run over and, of course, life happens, but I try to make sure that at least 3–4 times during the day I am up and about moving in some way. Having a standing desk has also changed my life, and I highly recommend getting one if it works with what you do.

If you work in an office or away from home, find ways to have mini movement breaks that are practical and realistic based on your working conditions. It could be walking up and down the stairs at work, heading outside and walking around the building, or around the block if you have time. If there is a chance to stand up and walk around when you are taking a call, that can work, too, and you can see if you can get a standing desk. Even doing a few squats in the bathroom when you are there can work! Anything that gets you moving. Walking meetings are also a super idea, and something I try to do whenever it is practical.

Chapter 11
Relationships

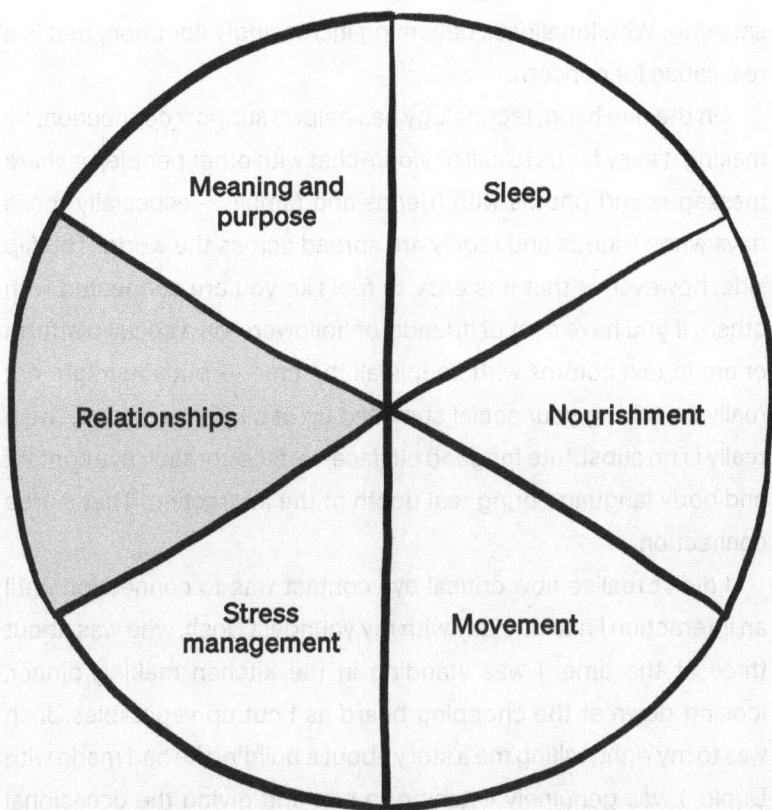

Meaning and purpose

Sleep

Relationships

Nourishment

Stress management

Movement

When it comes to conversations about relationships and wellbeing, we need to consider both our relationships with others *and* our relationship with ourselves.

First and foremost, we are a social species. Historically, the survival of our species depended on us being part of a group. If you struck out alone, you were very likely to die. As such, the need for social connection is hard-wired into the systems in our brains and is necessary to help us feel safe.

That doesn't mean, though, that you need to be 'in a relationship', or love spending lots of time talking to people, or be a super-social person. It simply means that none of us evolved to spend a lot of time on our own without interacting with other people. So much so that evidence now suggests that loneliness is as bad for you as smoking. With loneliness becoming increasingly common, that is a real cause for concern.

On the one hand, technology has helped support connection, by making it easy for us to call or video-chat with other people, or share messages and photos with friends and family — especially these days when friends and family are spread across the world. The flip side, however, is that it is easy to *feel* like you are connected with others if you have a lot of 'friends' or 'followers' on a social platform or are in text comms with people all the time — but you might not really be having your social cup filled up at all. To be honest, there really is no substitute for good old face-to-face contact; eye contact and body language bring real depth to the interaction. That is true connection.

I didn't realise how critical eye contact was to connection until an interaction I had one day with my youngest, Josh, who was about three at the time. I was standing in the kitchen making dinner, looking down at the chopping board as I cut up vegetables. Josh was to my right, telling me a story about a building he had made with Duplo. I was genuinely listening to him and giving the occasional verbal response, but after about a minute he stamped his foot and grabbed my arm and said, in his three-year-old English, 'You not listening.'

I replied that I *was* listening, and repeated what he had just told me, but he wasn't having a bar of it. 'You not listening because you not looking at me,' he shouted.

Wow. It really hit me that sometimes little kids know so much more than adults. While, yes, I was listening, what Josh was trying to say was that I wasn't really *engaging*. He wasn't getting the social cues from me that he needed to feel we were having a real human interaction. These cues — facial expressions and body language — are how children learn the social 'rules' of interaction. Without adequate interaction of this type, children can develop dysfunctional behaviours, and this is something we are seeing being more and more of in our modern world.

When we are looking at our phones while talking to children, we have to remember: **our words alone are not enough as a response**. Children need to see our eyes and see our expressions change. This has been one of the most useful things I have ever learnt, and it has certainly made it easier for me to put a barrier between myself and my phone now I know the true cost.

While it is not possible to give all your attention to others all the time, this experience made me realise how fragmented so many of our social interactions can be these days. Phones on the tables at dinnertime are picked up immediately there's a notification. I'm sure we've all been in an online meeting with someone who is clearly reading other emails and responding to them at the same time. You can tell that your friend, colleague or family member is scrolling on their phone while you are trying to talk to them. Many of us watch TV while having dinner together ... the list goes on. It just isn't good.

One thing I distinctly notice about the Blue Zone areas in the world that I mentioned earlier (see page 159) is how fundamental good relationships are. The people in these cultures spend time together; they talk together, dance together, sit together, cook together, eat together. It is something so simple, yet so profound when it comes to wellbeing.

What social connection will look like for you will be different from what it looks like for me, and different for others you know, but I felt it imperative to include this conversation in this book because human connection is so essential for mental and physical wellbeing. Also, when you feel disconnected or lonely, or other difficult emotions arise as a result of poor-quality connections, food and drink can become a stand-in for connection or act as a distraction, which is something I see so often.

I recommend that you look at how you can be more truly connected with others. That might mean addressing your relationship with your phone, or having a conversation with others in your life about *their* phone usage. (Good luck if you do that — I know it is not an easy one.)

Beyond phones and other devices, the way to go might be locking in a regular weekly or monthly catch-up with a group of friends for a walk, some sport, a meal or a bike ride. Or reconnecting with an old hobby that encourages you to connect face to face with others who have a similar interest. Maybe it is time to trade your home gym for a real gym, something I have recently done myself.

Animals can have an amazing presence, too; you'll know this already if you have a pet. I never had a pet growing up, but since reading the research on how pets improve your wellbeing, we recently welcomed a cute wee dog to our family — and it really has been amazing. I know pets aren't for everyone, but they can be another tool to consider if you are experiencing loneliness. Do, however, make sure you have the time and resources to look after one.

'Wherever you are, be all there.'

— missionary Jim Elliot

Your relationship with yourself

When I was going through therapy in my twenties, one question I was asked by the psychologist was: 'What do you consider your relationship with yourself to be like?' I didn't really know what she meant, so I had to ask for clarification.

She told me that my relationship with myself was how I thought and felt about myself. She also wanted to know how well I looked after myself.

I sat for a while and allowed what she said to land, because back then I had only ever thought about relationships in terms of the interactions I had with friends, family and who I worked with; never that I somehow had a relationship with myself.

Finally, I replied that I didn't really like myself. In fact, much of the time when I was younger I really hated myself, and I didn't really think that my life was worth much to anyone. In terms of looking after myself, other than saying I did exercise and ate okay, I didn't really know what else to say.

Saying this out loud for the first time in this way really struck me. Despite getting high grades in my A levels (equivalent to NCEA 3 or Bursary) and coming second in the year in my full-time degree, how come I had never before come across this concept of having a relationship with myself? Might it help me change the way I felt about myself?

are, be all there.

— Alsacnery I a Eliot

KEY MESSAGE

Be a good companion to yourself — you have to live with yourself forever.

Your relationship with yourself

When I was doing the 12th method in my exercise, one question

The floodgates were open and I did a deep dive of exploration into the topic. (A common theme in this book now — my deep dives after breakdowns and revelations!)

The concept of understanding yourself, knowing *why* you are who you are, *why* you think how you think, *why* you do what you do and *why* certain patterns in your life keep repeating themselves has become my uppermost passion. It drew me to study positive psychology because a huge part of that study was learning about your relationships with others and with yourself.

You are with you forever, so learning about yourself, and learning to like yourself, respect yourself and maybe even love yourself can truly be one of life's biggest gifts. If you can learn to give yourself the love you give to others, forgive yourself for your mistakes and screw-ups, and be compassionate towards yourself for all that you have been through, it can give you freedom like nothing else. You aren't perfect. But you aren't meant to be. You are HUMAN, after all.

So often in life we are waiting for someone to accept us, for someone to deeply and truly understand us — but really, **what we**

need to do first is understand and accept *ourselves* so we don't end up chasing validation and acceptance from others.

In Chapter 1, we looked at your iceberg in relation to the way you think and feel about your body and the way you eat. Now, we will take it one step further and look in more detail at some of the other aspects in the hidden part of the iceberg: your beliefs, values and thoughts. We will also revisit emotions to see how addressing these can help you have a better relationship with yourself.

Beliefs

To save you flicking back through the pages, here is a mini recap on beliefs:

- Your beliefs are assumptions you have about yourself, the world and other people.
- You don't consciously choose your beliefs as a child, but they develop as a way for your brain to make sense of the information it receives from the world around you as you are growing up. In a way, your beliefs are a form of self-protection.
- Your beliefs essentially become part of the rule book by which you subconsciously make decisions in your life, and can influence both your relationship with yourself and your relationship with others.
- Your beliefs can be helpful — or they can be unhelpful, also known as 'limiting' beliefs. These are the ones that can trigger a chain reaction of negative self-talk, eroding your worth and self-esteem and negatively impacting the direction of your life.

- Your core beliefs are the statements that you believe to be completely true about yourself. These statements often start with the word 'I' — for example, 'I am confident' or 'I am unlovable'.
- Core beliefs can then get supporting beliefs tacked on to them. For example: 'I am confident' — *I can do anything I put my mind to*. 'I am unlovable' — *I will be alone forever*.
- Your beliefs can impact your thoughts, and your thoughts can impact your beliefs.

To help you understand how beliefs develop, first up I will use my life as an example. Then . . . it will be time to think about yours!

As a child, I felt like if I disappeared then no one would miss me. I fundamentally believed I was broken, because at primary school no one wanted to be around me and even if they did it wasn't okay to tell others. I distinctly remember one girl whose mum was friends with my mum. On Thursdays, I went to her house after school until I could be picked up by my mum, who worked late those days. I loved it. We had a great time playing together and I felt like I had a real friend for the first time. But there was a downside; a big one. At school, she had to pretend she wasn't friends with me because otherwise her other friends wouldn't talk to her — because, to all the other kids, I was a bit weird.

I formed a *limiting belief* that I wasn't good enough, and in hindsight this kicked off the destruction of the relationship I had with myself. Even when I did manage to make friends later on, part of me always believed it was temporary. My limiting belief then led me to constantly seek validation from others to help prove that maybe, somehow, I was worthy enough to be with them. This belief led me to swear a lot to try to look 'cool', and act up and tell stupid jokes to get a positive reaction from my peers. It also led me to look in other places for validation, like controlling my food and study endlessly.

Counting my calories and sticking to a plan somehow made me feel like I was at least good at *something*. Being near the top of the class made me feel validated at school and helped soften the blow of feeling like I didn't belong. This limiting belief continued through senior school, university and into the early years of my working life — until I finally learnt about beliefs and the impact they can have.

I then did the work to change this limiting belief, or, to be more realistic, soften it a little, and it worked: this has helped me improve how I think and feel about myself. That work primarily involves breaking down the belief and seeing if it really is 100% true, or if it is, indeed, just something you have come to believe is true when it is not. This is an exercise I will be taking you through soon.

Doing the work to reprogram a belief doesn't mean it will be gone forever. I am always aware of my limiting beliefs, and they still rear their ugly heads at times, but overall I have much more control over them than before. You can be much more in control of yours, too.

As well as the many limiting beliefs I developed, I also had lots of positive ones! My parents always encouraged me to just 'do my best' and not worry about the outcome. They taught me that I didn't need to win, I didn't need to be the best, I didn't need to compare my work to others. As long as I gave everything a go and always gave it my best effort, that was good enough. I am so grateful for this being drilled into me as a child because now I have the confidence to give *anything* a go, even if I really suck at it; because it is about trying new things and giving your best, not about needing to be the best.

————————

What parts of your own past are playing out now for you? What are the limiting beliefs that are holding you back? How can you rework your narrative to create better beliefs that lead you in the direction of your dreams to create a life you love?

What are your beliefs?

A simple way to work out what you believe is by answering the following questions. Write as many words as feels right next to each one. Avoid thinking too hard about this — just trust what your gut tells you and write down what first comes to mind. I know you might think, *Claire, I don't have time to do this now*, but trust me: you don't have the time in your life not to. Being aware of what you believe and seeing how this is affecting your life is major, and has the ability to positively impact the trajectory of your life.

I am . . .

The world is . . .

Other people are . . .

The table on the opposite page gives some examples to get you started. Instead of writing them down, you could circle any that feel like they fit you, and add more of your own.

Then look at the lists you wrote down or the beliefs you circled.

- How do these beliefs make you feel?
- Do other people you know have similar views?
- Can you stop any limiting beliefs? Ones that might be holding you back from being your best in life or might be sabotaging you somehow.
- It is time to interrogate your limiting beliefs! Are these beliefs 100% true? If you think to yourself, *yep, totally true*, I want you to think of it like this: could you argue in a court of law, as if your life depended on it, that these beliefs are actually, in all circumstances, without a doubt 100% true? If you can see that maybe it is not 100% true, how true is it really? 70%? 50%? 30%?

Beliefs about yourself	Beliefs about the world	Beliefs about other people
Capable	The world is inherently a good place.	Most people are inherently good.
Resilient		
Deserving of happiness	There is plenty for everyone in the world.	People can change if they are given the chance.
In control of my life	Change is possible.	There are people around to help me.
Valuable	Progress is possible.	I can count on other people.
Worthy of respect	Human beings are all connected.	
Worthy of forgiveness	There is hope for the future.	I can trust most people.
Compassionate		I am loved by others.
Authentic	The world is dangerous.	People I love always leave me.
Connected	Life is not fair.	
Too old	The way the world is makes life hard.	You can't count on other people.
Too big	The world is stacked against me.	Other people are out to get me.
Busy		
Weak	The future is hopeless.	People will always let you down.
Out of control	The world is full of injustice.	People only care about themselves.
Needy		
Trapped		It is not safe to trust other people.
A failure		
Not good enough		
Unlovable		
Unattractive		
Likely to be rejected		
Likely to be abandoned		
Likely to be alone		
Different from other people		
Worthless		
Bad		
Immoral		
Boring		

A key thing to understand about beliefs is that, without us realising, over time our beliefs get stronger and stronger. They act a bit like magnets — they attract evidence from our experiences and the world around us to back up what we believe, repelling anything that might challenge them.

This can, in fact, be helpful. Say you have the helpful belief that 'it is worth giving everything a try'. You will likely look for opportunities and evidence that support the benefits of trying new things, rather than looking for evidence that trying new things can be negative, like being expensive, or a waste of time, or a distraction.

It can also be *unhelpful*. For example, if you believe that you aren't good at making friends and no one wants to spend time with you, how do you interpret this situation: *You are at the supermarket and a lady you have met a couple of times before walks past you without acknowledging you.* That can only mean that she doesn't like you, right? Or that you have done something wrong? Did you say something bad the last time you saw her? Maybe you aren't her kind of person? Maybe you aren't anyone's kind of person? . . . Your head goes into a spin.

You collected evidence to support a belief you have about yourself. But there are all sorts of other explanations for what happened that could be equally true. One is that she just didn't see you! (This happens to me all the time, as I can't see well without my glasses, and I am sure I often unintentionally ignore people I know when I don't have my specs on.) Maybe she had a bad day and didn't feel like talking to anyone — maybe it was nothing to do with you at all.

This sort of thing is why we really need to question our beliefs as to how true they really are, because our default view on this is likely to be very skewed.

Reworking limiting beliefs

I use a three-step process to rework the narrative for my limiting beliefs. Here is how it works:

STEP 1: You need to collect evidence AGAINST this limiting belief; evidence that exists in the here and now.

You might feel like your belief is 100% true, but when you really look at it deeply, there will be all sorts of evidence that doesn't align with it.

Example: I have no confidence.

Yes, you might lack confidence when you meet new people. But do you lack confidence with your mum? Your brother/sister? Your dog? The person at the supermarket counter? Are you lacking confidence 100% of the time? Or maybe just 80% of the time?

You need to see that this *isn't* 100% who you are. Know that over time, that 80% can be dialled down if you BELIEVE it can be.

STEP 2: What is a better belief that is more aligned with who you are today and who you want to show up as in the world?

Write this down. Write it on a Post-It note and put it on your mirror. Repeat it multiple times, morning and night. Help this belief become part of you. This is so important!

Example: I can be confident.

STEP 3: Look for *evidence to support your new belief.*

Start to notice when things happen that align with the belief you are trying to build. If you can, put yourself in situations where you will be able to *create* evidence that this new belief is true.

Example: I looked another person in the eyes when I was walking down the street and actually smiled at them rather than looking at the ground.

Example: I shared an idea in a team meeting today.

―――――

I will be honest: this process does take work, and it does take time — but it can change your life forever. What I have given you here is a snapshot of the basics. If you can see that this is something you need to do more focused work on, reach out to a qualified registered psychologist or psychotherapist to support you through the process.

Trauma and beliefs

It is important to acknowledge the effect of trauma on beliefs, as this can significantly distort and strengthen the power of the false and limiting beliefs.

Children rely on their caregivers for survival and for the basic needs of food, water and shelter, so if children are treated badly or something bad happens, as I mentioned earlier (see page 127), it is safer for them to believe that *they* are the cause of the problems rather than believing that the people looking after them are responsible.

Likewise, if things go wrong in the world around them, be that a natural disaster or a change in their living situation, it can be easy for children to create the belief that they are to blame for what's happened. These beliefs can then shape their lives forever unless the work is done to change them. They can create invisible walls through trying to manage deep wounds.

Trauma can also be experienced beyond the childhood years in so many ways — living through natural disasters, car crashes, losing loved ones, relationship breakdowns, divorce, emotional abuse, physical abuse, chronic illnesses, financial issues, job losses ... and so the list goes on.

If you have experienced trauma, see my suggestions for further reading under 'Trauma' in the resources section on page 296.

Values

Part of my study in positive psychology involved a deep dive into understanding values. Values are the things that really matter to us — from belonging, to commitment, to power, to loyalty and everything in between.

One day my classmates and I completed an activity which has changed my life forever. We were asked to lay out a pack of cards, each of which had a word on it which reflected a core value. We had to look at all the cards and pick the top ten that stood out as being the most important to us. The ten things that felt like they deeply mattered and, if it came to it, we would be willing to risk our lives for.

It was hard to do. There were so many good values there, but after a while it became clear that some were far more important than others.

We were *then* asked to go back through our ten and get rid of five of them. For the remaining cards, the five most important values, we were to rank them from top to bottom.

For me it was ...

1. Belonging
2. Kindness
3. Adventure
4. Service
5. Growth

A light bulb went off in my head! Looking at my five words, I could understand why my life had turned out the way it had. I could clearly see what had driven me to make the choices I had made — sometimes to my benefit, other times to my detriment. I could also see why I struggle to connect with some people; we just have really opposed values. And I saw why so many arguments with my husband were just going around in circles: while some of our values align, others really don't!

When you are living a life that allows you to be in line with what you value, you are likely to feel more contented, calmer, and like you 'fit' into your world. It can make you doubt yourself less, feel better about yourself, and be more confident to embrace your own authenticity.

When you are living a life that is *not* aligned with your values, however, it can feel like you are walking through deep mud on your own much of the time, just trying to get through, push on. It can feel that you need to shout to be heard, but even so, no one seems to listen.

Once you become aware of what your core values are, you will start to see why you behave and react the way you do and what has driven you to make many of the choices you have made in your life. You can also start to make more informed choices about what you do in the future, based on what aligns with your values and what doesn't.

What are your core values?

Do the same exercise I did: look at this list (it continues overleaf) and circle your top ten. Then highlight your top five, and rank them.

accountability	confidence	financial stability
achievement	connection	forgiveness
adaptability	contentment	freedom
adventure	contribution	friendship
altruism	cooperation	fun
ambition	courage	future generations
authenticity	creativity	generosity
balance	curiosity	giving back
beauty	dignity	grace
being the best	diversity	gratitude
belonging	efficiency	growth
career	environment	harmony
caring	equality	health
collaboration	ethics	home
commitment	excellence	honesty
community	fairness	hope
compassion	faith	humility
competence	family	humour

inclusion	parenting	simplicity
independence	patience	spirituality
initiative	patriotism	sportsmanship
integrity	peace	stewardship
intuition	perseverance	success
job security	personal fulfilment	teamwork
joy	power	thrift
justice	pride	time
kindness	recognition	tradition
knowledge	reliability	travel
leadership	resourcefulness	trust
learning	respect	truth
legacy	responsibility	understanding
leisure	risk-taking	uniqueness
love	safety	usefulness
loyalty	security	vision
making a difference	self-discipline	vulnerability
nature	self-expression	wealth
openness	self-respect	wellbeing
optimism	serenity	wholeheartedness
order	service	wisdom

Having identified your values, the next step is to reflect on how much your life is currently in line with them. This is not something that can be done in five minutes while reading this section — it is something to ponder on over the coming days, weeks and months.

My suggestion is to write down your top five values and put them somewhere you will see them every day — in your diary, on your fridge, on your desk, on your screen-saver, whatever works.

As you reflect, also think about what you could do and what decisions you could make to help you feel like you are living more in line with your values.

For me, with *belonging* I have consciously made decisions in my life that enhance my sense of having a community around me. This is one of the reasons that Mission Nutrition exists. I also choose to work in a shared office sometimes despite it being more expensive than working from home, because to feel like myself I need a 'work family'.

Kindness is at the core of many of my decisions. I intentionally spread kindness to others, carry out random acts of kindness, and read or engage with podcasts that are about kindness. I also have to consciously distance myself from people who are unkind and have no interest in being any different.

With *adventure*, I need to be outside, and I also need to be trying new things. This hadn't happened much in the years leading up to writing this book and it was a core reason why I ended up relocating — so that I could feel more like myself with the easy access to adventures and the opportunity to try new things in a new place.

For *service*, this is why I am here. Why I have given up long weekends and (temporarily) time with my family to be here for you and to do what I do because it is something I value highly; it is fundamental to me feeling like my life is worth living. My work is my service. I am driven to make a difference in other people's lives. The win for me is that doing this for work makes me feel like myself because it is in line with what I value.

Lastly, *growth*. If I am not learning new things, trying new things or being challenged mentally, I feel totally lost. It is why I have a business coach, why I tried karate in my forties, and why I plan to take up pottery and mountain biking. It is why I read, listen and learn as much as I can.

Despite the challenges I still continue to face in my life, I feel so much more like myself and make decisions that feel in line with who I am now, simply because I know what my values are and I let these be my compass.

I said it before, and I will say it again: **Knowing your values has the potential to change your life.**

Your thoughts

Your thoughts are essentially the conversation you have with yourself day in, day out. It is a bit like having a commentator living in your head who is constantly giving you feedback on things that happened in the past, what might happen in the future, or what is happening right now. An internal monologue, if you like.

These thoughts combined with your beliefs and biases are known as your 'self-talk'. Some of this self-talk will be about you, some of it is about other people, and some won't have anything to do with people at all.

Most of us aren't really that in tune with our self-talk; we might only become aware of it sometimes when we are sitting on our own, or are going into a situation that makes us feel uncomfortable. However, for some of us our self-talk will feel like it is very loud, much of the time.

The critical thing to understand when it comes to your self-talk is that just because you think something in your head *that doesn't always make it true*. Yes, if you see a black cat and think, *that is a black cat*, this is indeed true — but what about thoughts like, *I can't do this, I won't do well, I will always be single, I don't deserve to be happy*? Are those actually true? 100% true?

Like unhelpful beliefs, your thoughts need to be questioned because they can, sneakily, cause you to create a story about yourself that you *make* true because you believe it to be — not because it *is* true.

When you need a reminder that you are *not* your thoughts, imagine yourself on one side of a line (I have drawn a picture of this for my kids). On the other side are your thoughts, your friends, what you eat and drink, how much money you earn, where you live and so on. You do not have to be defined by any of these things!

Here are a couple of examples of thoughts in action and how unhelpful self-talk can play out:

- You get annoyed with your friend for constantly going on about a guy you both know she shouldn't date, but who she continues to contact daily, and you find yourself thinking, *honestly, she knows better, why does she always do this?* Does it make you a bad friend just because you thought that? No. That, along with your other thoughts, is just part of you processing the situation. When you are with your friend, you will most likely keep those thoughts to yourself knowing that she is your bestie and you will be there no matter what. Or, equally, you might choose at some point to share your thoughts, but in a gentler way that will be more helpful for getting your point across.
- Every time you look in the mirror, you think to yourself, *I am unattractive*. That thought being repetitive doesn't make it true. It might be based on a belief that is cemented in your head because as a child you always felt like you were less attractive than your sister or your friends. But it doesn't

ACTUALLY mean that you are indeed unattractive. The thought is likely to make you devalue yourself, not want to look after yourself, not smile, not dress in the way that makes you feel more confident, not bother to get your hair done in a way that makes you feel good — confirming to yourself that you aren't attractive.

Negative self-talk can end up creating self-fulfilling prophecies. If you think you are no good at something, let's say cooking, it will likely go badly and then you have proved yourself right. You have attracted evidence to prove what you think and believe to be true. Such a trap!

If, instead, you go in with the thoughts, *I am new to cooking, I need to give myself time to learn, that was a good first effort and I learnt a thing or two*, you will change the game for yourself.

What is your self-talk like?

As with getting to understand your behaviours and your beliefs, the only way to change negative self-talk and negative thinking is to first become aware of the patterns that you might not really be in tune with.

Keeping a daily journal for a few weeks can be a useful starting point to help you become more aware of your thinking patterns and any limiting beliefs. You could write for two minutes a day, or an hour if you want to and have the time. Highlight any thoughts you pick up that are unhelpful or unkind — the ones you are saying to yourself but would never say to your friend, a child, your pet or someone else you love.

If sitting down and journalling every day doesn't work for you, you can just capture negative thoughts as they come up in real time throughout the day. Whatever is realistic and practical for you can become a daily habit.

Writing is *such* a powerful tool. There is a reason I encourage you to put pen to paper so many times in this book. It is free, and it works.

Mindfulness and meditation practices can support you to become more aware of your thoughts. The critical thing to remember, though, is not to judge the thoughts when you notice them; they are only thoughts, after all. Just be aware that they are there, knowing that you *do* have the power to change the ones that are negatively impacting your life.

After a week or two, find time to sit down quietly and reflect on what you have written. What are the patterns? What are the helpful and constructive thoughts? What are the repetitive negative or dysfunctional thoughts?

Once you have awareness of some of the negative thoughts you are having, it is a great practice to give these thoughts a name, a label or a character (like you did with your unhelpful habits). This helps you to separate the thoughts from you as a person. An example might be calling these thoughts your inner gremlin, inner critic, fire thoughts . . . whatever works for you!

This character is the part of you that feeds the negative self-talk — it is NOT who you are. Your job in building a healthier relationship with yourself is to tame this gremlin, critic or fire-starter! **You are here to run the show now, *not* those default, automatic, unhelpful, destructive thoughts.**

Addressing your thinking is SUCH an important part of your journey to creating a healthier relationship with food, your body and yourself. You need thoughts that support your journey rather than drive you away from the path you want to go on. Living your life with negative self-talk in charge might feel normal to you, but it is not helpful.

_____

Instead of letting our negative thoughts run the show, firstly we need to challenge them: are they really true? Secondly, we need to replace them with neutral or positive thoughts. Here's how this worked for me when it came to writing this book.

When I was initially approached to write the book, I was excited. I got my concept and plan together, agreed it with the publisher and then, with my go-getter attitude, cracked into getting it done as soon as possible.

It wasn't long before my negative self-talk kicked in, though:

- *Who am I to write a book like this?*
- *I am qualified in positive psychology, but I am not a fully-fledged psychologist — I will get torn apart. What if I say something that isn't right without knowing?*
- *Other nutritionists will pick me to bits; some won't agree with what I say.*
- *I don't have a PhD; all the good podcasters and authors right now are also scientists, doing research. I don't know what they know.*
- *What if people don't like what I say?*
- *What if what I write doesn't make sense?*
- *I really find writing hard. It is not my natural strength. I always was terrible at spelling at school. I have only read one paper book in my life because I struggle to read with my type of dyslexia.*

This self-talk went on and on. Day after day, every time I sat down to write, every night before bed, every time I talked about it, thought about it, up these negative thoughts would come.

As I became aware of this negative self-talk, I discussed it with my business coach and recognised that it was time to challenge these thoughts and replace them with neutral or positive thoughts. Here's how that went . . .

- *Who am I to write a book like this?*
  Challenge the thought: *Anyone is entitled to have a go at writing a book.*
  New thought: *People need this book — if I don't write this, who will help them?*
- *I am qualified in positive psychology, but I am not a fully-fledged psychologist — I will get torn apart. What if I say something that isn't right without knowing?*
  Challenge the thought: *It is not 100% true that I will get torn apart.*
  New thoughts: *I am not claiming to be a psychologist, and I will get my work peer-reviewed. If some people disagree with what I say, that is okay; but for most people it will be helpful.*
- *Other nutritionists will pick me to bits; some won't agree with what I say.*
  Challenge the thought: *Some might pick me apart; most won't.*
  New thought: *With 20 years of personal and professional experience behind me, I am entitled to share my point of view.*
- *I don't have a PhD; all the good podcasters and authors right now are also scientists, doing research. I don't know what they know.*
  Challenge the thought: *Yes, there are more and more researchers writing and speaking, and they are great, but there are plenty of other people who don't have PhDs who*

also do amazing work. It is not 100% true that I need to have a PhD to write a good book.
New thought: *I am doing the best I can with what I know, and am making that clear to my readers.*

- *What if people don't like what I say?*
Challenge the thought: *Some won't, but that isn't the majority. So there is not enough evidence to stop me writing a book.*
New thought: *Some people will really connect with what I am saying and it could make a real difference to them.*

- *What if what I write doesn't make sense?*
Challenge the thought: *There are fully qualified editors and a great team of publishers who will make sure it makes sense.*
New thought: *I will do my best writing, and that is good enough.*

- *I really find writing hard. It is not my natural strength. I always was terrible at spelling at school. I have only read one paper book in my life because I struggle to read with my type of dyslexia.*
Challenge the thought: *Not everyone who writes books has the same level of skill.*
New thought: *Writing is hard, but I have done it before so I can do it again.*

This is a process you can go through with your own thoughts at any time. It is normal to have negative thoughts, but the goal is to tip the balance so you don't allow them to take over your life.

As well as reframing your negative thoughts, consciously choosing to add positive thoughts into your head is also incredibly helpful.

This can be done in many ways.

You can create the ritual of standing in front of the mirror in the morning and repeating positive statements to yourself over and over until they become new beliefs. Things like 'I am capable', 'I can do this', and 'I deserve to feel joy in my life'. If the mirror feels like a bit too much to start with, try doing it in your head for the first few minutes after you get up in the morning — before you grab your phone!

One thing I find particularly helpful for reframing my thinking throughout the day is having great quotes or affirmations where I can see them. On my office wall I have 'She believed she could, so she did'. On my fridge I have 'There are a lot of things to be grateful for'. The screen-saver on my computer says 'You are capable of amazing things'. I also bought my friend a bracelet that says 'Wake up, kick arse, be kind, repeat'. She wears is every day. There are so many different quotes out there — find ones that work for you.

'If you own this story you get to write the ending.'

— researcher and storyteller Brené Brown

Self-compassion

Would you shout at a child for not tying their shoelaces properly in their first week of learning this new skill?

Would you call your best friend fat and lazy if she gained weight and couldn't do her jeans up?

Would you tell a colleague who you really get on with and respect that there is no chance they will get the promotion they are going for because they aren't good or smart enough?

No. You wouldn't.

So why is it okay that we do this to ourselves? If it wouldn't work for a child or our friends, why would it ever work for us? If being hard on yourself worked, it would have done so by now! Spoiler alert: it doesn't work.

Alongside noticing our negative thoughts, reframing them and practising adding positive thoughts into the mix, we also need to practise the skill of **self-compassion** to help beat our negative self-talk. Yep: this is a *skill*, something you can learn which can become a habit.

A simple way to start doing it is this: when you catch your negative self-talk in action, think to yourself one of these three things; whichever feels right for you:

- How would I talk to a friend in this situation?
- What would I say to a child right now?
- What would I want someone to say to me as a child if I was thinking/feeling this?

'You deserve the love and compassion you so freely give to others.'

— Unknown source

Another excellent thing to do to foster self-compassion is to write down five things you like about yourself. If your self-talk has a strong negative skew, I know this might be really challenging. If it feels too hard, write down five nice things that someone else you know would say about you, or even five things your pet would want you to know. (They mostly like think you're pretty darn awesome!)

I encourage you to explore this further if it feels like an area you need to work on. Many of the meditation and mindfulness practices you come across on apps like Calm, Headspace and Insight Timer include some form of self-compassion practice, so rest assured that there are many tools out there. Dr Kristin Neff is an expert in this area, so you can look her up, too!

The impact of others

A core theme in this book has been looking at the hidden part of your iceberg to see how your beliefs, values, thoughts, habits and emotions affect the way you behave. Just for a moment, however,

I want to put the spotlight on how other people behave and how what is going on for them in their iceberg might be negatively affecting you.

Have you come across people in your life who always put you down? Or people who try to put their problems onto you? People who are nice to you, then in the next breath say something unkind or hurtful? This is the unhelpful invisible stuff in their own iceberg coming out, being projected at you (and no doubt towards other people in their lives). I have come across so many people in my life like this, who despite some positive traits seem to be constantly looking to bring others down.

If this has happened or is happening to you, please know that it has got *nothing* to do with you and *everything* to do with them.

The simple fact is that 'hurt people hurt other people'. The internal struggle they are having with themselves is coming out because they haven't learnt the skills or tools to manage what is going on inside.

When my kids get picked on at school, I remind them of this. Bullies or people who are mean to you in any way are simply those who are struggling with themselves, who are trying to make themselves feel better by bringing other people down. Their motive is to numb their own pain; it is just that you get caught up in the process.

I constantly have to remind myself and my adult friends of this, too. One friend has a very challenging woman in her workplace who is always trying to get one up on her and do anything she can to bring my friend down. But this has nothing to do with my friend, and everything to do with the pain and sadness this other woman is feeling on the inside, being projected in a toxic, cruel way. After talking through this with me, my friend is no longer taking things personally, and if this is happening in your life then you shouldn't either.

'You can't control what other people think about you, but you can control how you think about yourself.'

— Unknown source

Notice the good

As I noted in Chapter 7, on sleep, we have a natural negative bias which means we are drawn to focus more on the bad than the good in our lives. This negative bias can drive our negative thinking and negative self-talk and result in us feeling negative about our lives.

An example of this is what happens when your head hits the pillow at night. Do you think to yourself how nice it was that a random stranger helped you get a trolley in the supermarket? Or how nice the email was from your boss today? Or how well your kids emptied the dishwasher? No, you probably don't think of any of that. Instead, you are likely to replay all the negative things that happened in your day. The guy who took your car parking place. The toast you burnt this morning. The insurance bill you got that has increased by 30%.

Both the positive and the negative things really happened, but your mind latches on to the negative ones and replays them over and over in preference to the positive.

To help balance this out, we have to notice that it's happening. As always, **awareness** is the first stage of change. Then consciously **practise** noticing the good; another healthy habit to cultivate.

When you go to bed at night, focus on the things that went well that day, to tell your brain a new story. Pick a number of things to focus on. It might be three, five, ten, or whatever works for you and allows this practice to become a habit. Including things you are grateful for can also be part of this practice. The research to support the benefits of gratitude is incredible. It really works.

When this has become a strong habit at night, you will hopefully then be able to catch yourself during the day, too, when you are getting caught in the trap of noticing all the problems. Even on the most difficult of days, look at what is working; something good, however small, is likely to have happened. Even just having a nice cup of tea in the morning or taking a warm shower.

Research by Dr Barbara Fredrickson suggests that in order to experience optimal wellbeing, creativity and success, we need to maintain a 3:1 ratio of positive to negative emotions. This means that for every negative thought or emotion, we need three positive ones to balance this out. Something to keep top of mind to support your wellbeing.

'You can't hate yourself into a version of someone that you love.'
— author Lori Deschene

Chapter 12
Meaning and purpose

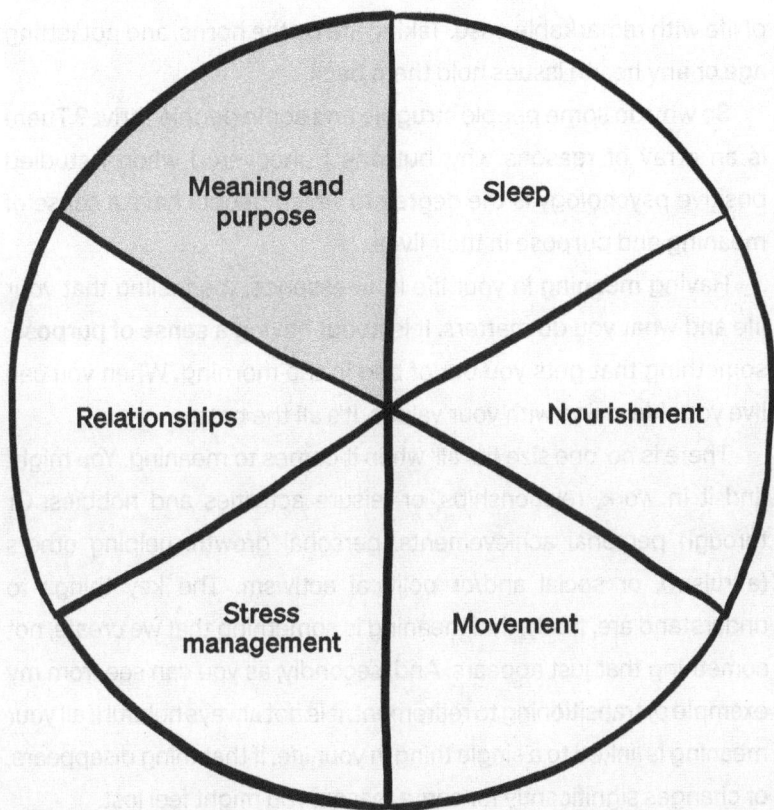

Something I've seen over and over again is just how differently people manage the transition between their working life and retirement.

Some people really struggle. They find it hard to figure out who they are, and what life is about on the other side of being defined by their work. The same can happen for those who have children, both when they become parents and also when the kids all leave home. There can be a sense of loss, which might show up as depression or some other mental health challenge. It is hard to watch.

Other people flourish when they have more time and freedom, and can't seem to remember how they possibly ever had time to work. My mum and dad are these kinds of people. More than anyone I have ever known or met, they have transitioned to their new phase of life with remarkable ease. Taking life by the horns, and not letting age or any health issues hold them back.

So why do some people struggle and some people thrive? There is an array of reasons why, but one I uncovered when I studied positive psychology is the degree to which people have a sense of meaning and purpose in their lives.

Having **meaning** in your life is, in essence, the feeling that your life and what you do *matters*. It is about having a **sense of purpose**, something that gets you out of bed in the morning. When you can live your life in line with your values, it's all the better.

There is no 'one size fits all' when it comes to meaning. You might find it in work, relationships, or leisure activities and hobbies. Or through personal achievements, personal growth, helping others (altruism), or social and/or political activism. The key things to understand are, firstly, that meaning is something that we *create*, not something that just appears. And, secondly, as you can see from my example of transitioning to retirement, it is not always helpful if all your meaning is linked to a single thing in your life. If that thing disappears, or changes significantly for some reason, you might feel lost.

My parents transitioned easily into retirement because as well as having a sense of meaning in their lives from their work and from being parents to my brothers and me, they also had things outside of this which they were able to continue when work was gone and we were, too.

My grandmother was a music teacher, so my dad has always had musical interests. He has always been part of a choir and played the piano since he was a child. When he retired he also took up the double bass and now plays in an orchestra. Through the ups and downs of his cancer treatment over the past few years, music has given him a sense of purpose and a reason to get out of bed in the morning. I genuinely believe that his love for music and being part of choirs and an orchestra have been a huge part of why he continues to hold hope while fighting for his survival.

My mum grew up on a farm and has always had a keen interest in gardening and where food comes from. Come rain or shine, she is outside tending to the vegetables and fruits that my parents grow, and when their crops are ready they enjoy the end of that journey by nourishing their bodies with the goodies they have grown.

Beyond their many personal interests, my parents are also part of many community groups. They have close friends, they support their elderly neighbours, they give their time to help others and get involved with many charity causes. They source meaning from many different things in their life.

You might be nowhere near having to think about retirement or life beyond your work or family years, but there are still many lessons in this story for all of us.

As part of your wellbeing tool kit, it is really important to reflect on what gives your life meaning. Research shows that people who have a higher sense of meaning and purpose in their lives are healthier, happier and live longer. In most of the Blue Zone cultures in the world, the cultures in which people live the longest, there are common phrases that describe the idea of purpose. In Okinawa, Japan, they call this *ikigai,* which translates to 'finding joy through purpose'. The Nicoyan people in Costa Rica use the phrase *plan de vida* or 'life plan' which they use in the sense of 'why I wake up in the morning'.

So, as well as sleeping well, eating well, keeping active, managing stress and having healthy relationships, this gem is something I really wanted to share with you in this small, but mighty, last chapter of the book.

Connecting with your meaning and purpose

You may already have a good sense of what matters to you and what drives you to get out of bed in the morning. But if you don't or are feeling lost right now, here are a few questions for you to ponder. You might not have answers for all of them; only some might resonate. Just explore what lands for *you.*

- If you were on your deathbed with only days to live, what three things would you have loved to have done with your life?
- What do you love to do?
- Is there anything you do where time feels like it passes by without you realising? Reading? Writing? Playing sport? Drawing? Singing?
- If you had the chance, what would you love to talk about or teach other people about all day?
- What are you extremely passionate about?
- What causes would you fight for?
- Where do you find the most inspiration?
- What have you accomplished that you are most proud of?

- What makes you feel like yourself when you do it?
- What makes you smile when you are doing it?
- What would you do if you knew you wouldn't fail?
- Is there a hobby or activity you have done in the past that you would really love to connect with again?
- Is there a way you can help other people?
- Is there something you can do to make the world a better place? Even if it is something tiny?

Having reflected on these questions, have a think about how your life right now lines up with the things that really matter to you. As you go through the coming days and weeks, you might see some opportunities to connect with things which give you a greater sense of meaning and purpose in your life. Especially if currently you are struggling in this space with your work and the other commitments you have.

Change and transition are normal parts of life, which means that at times we will likely face challenges connecting with our sense of meaning and purpose. We can't all give up our day jobs and pursue our hobbies or passions full-time, either. We can, however, get to know ourselves a bit better, work out what *meaning and purpose* means to us in our life in all its stages, and find a way to integrate things, however small, that make us feel like ourselves and that what we do matters.

As part of your exploration of meaning and purpose I encourage you to be open to trying new things — a new hobby, a craft, a musical instrument, a sport . . . I took up karate at 42 and was the only white belt in the room with every single one of the kids literally kicking my ass, but it has been a great way to open up my thinking and connect with other people.

If you have always wanted to try something, or recently got a buzz of interest for something but feel like you are too old or it is too late for that, let me tell you that it is NOT TOO LATE! My mum took up photography as a hobby when she retired; now, at age 74, she is winning photography competitions with her incredible work. From hardly knowing how to use a computer, she has taught herself Photoshop and other complicated editing programs and even prints her own photos! **It is *never* too late**.

TIME TO REFLECT: What one thing could you do to make you feel more aligned with who you really are? To make you feel more deeply connected to a sense of meaning and purpose?

Avoiding the 'success' trap

In our modern world, where having more money, more things and a higher status in our workplace are often portrayed as the ultimate goals, a trap we need to be aware of is the pursuit of 'more' being dressed up in the disguise of meaning and purpose.

While, yes, pushing yourself to reach society's definitions of success with a better job, car, house and so on can feel like you are winning, it often doesn't play out as the happy ending you might think it would. I have friends who are very wealthy and friends who just manage to pay their rent and always count their cents at the supermarket, and I can honestly tell you that, more often than not, the ones with more money aren't actually happier.

Of course, if you are struggling to meet your basic needs like food, water, clothing and shelter, more money *can* directly correlate with increased happiness, improved health and reduced stress. Once those needs are met, however, having a lot more money doesn't necessarily make you happier. When people get beyond a certain level of wealth, their happiness may actually start to decline. Wealth can cause a lot of problems, and some wealthy people have the most highly dysfunctional lives.

So yes: set your goals, reach for the stars, work hard and give life your all, but **do it for the right reasons** and be sure to check what your motivation for it is. Having a sense of meaning and purpose that makes you feel alive is so often found beyond the classic definition of success.

I have had to address this in my own life. In the past, my meaning and purpose was very much tied up in my work and it has been a slippery slope to manage that better. It is easy to want to chase the limelight and validation that can come with success at work, as well as the confirmation that you are doing 'well' because of all that you have achieved, but pushing yourself too hard in this direction has its consequences. It was undoubtedly part of my nervous system collapse. While my life in the past looked good on the outside, on the inside I often felt a sense of misalignment with myself.

I have since made some significant changes to my life. I realised that what really made me feel alive and made life worth living was being integrated in the lives of my close friends, knowing what they were up to, being able to support them when they were struggling, and feeling like we were a team in the crazy game of life. By working so hard to pursue 'success' at work, I had become disconnected from this other part of my life.

For me, meaning also comes from deeply connecting with my children. Not just sitting reading their schoolbooks with them at night while thinking about something else, but really being there, really showing up, looking them in the eye and connecting with them. This is something I haven't always done well.

Helping others has always given me meaning, too. While I do this in my work, I came to realise that I was no longer doing the charity work and other such activities that had been important in my life since I was a child. A disconnection to this part of me made me feel lost.

Understanding my meaning and purpose made me re-evaluate

many of the goals in my life. I set more manageable business goals, have consciously spent more time and energy connecting with my close friends, made space to be with my children and have engaged in more charity support activities.

This journey also made me re-assess my use of and engagement with social media. In the past, to help grow my businesses I had focused on growing my following, showing up every day to share the best of what I know, but in reality this was compromising other things I value in my life, like talking to my friends over dinner without taking photos of what we were eating, and making meals with my kids without having to video every step.

I realised that while I love sharing what I do with others on social media and know I can help other people this way, I needed to make sure it didn't take over my life to the degree that it was starting to. It was eroding my own wellbeing and the needs of my family and close friends, which is not an authentic representation of wellbeing!

Focusing instead on the connection with my kids and being a real friend to my closest crew has made so much difference. I really feel that my life is worth living.

The other part of the success trap to be aware of is that it encourages you to focus on the destination rather than the journey. But **the magic of life really is the journey** — it is the small moments among all the ups and downs which make life most special. When we get the 'thing' or reach the 'goal or target', it feels good for a while, but nowhere near as long as you think. The gloss soon wears off and you are left working towards the *next* big thing.

My hope for you as you reflect on your meaning and purpose is that you can start to get a sense of what really matters to you, what makes you feel alive and your life worth living, and can work to make more space for that in your life. When you are connected to what matters to you, you show up in the world as a better version of you, and this has a positive ripple effect on others.

Altruism

I believe it can be easy to overlook how much helping other people can improve our own wellbeing.

Altruism is the motivation to help another for the other person's benefit rather than our own. Opening the door for someone, letting someone go ahead of you in the supermarket queue, lifting someone's heavy bag up for them when they are struggling, or giving the last chocolate in the box to your friend.

Altruism is a vehicle through which we can introduce or enhance meaning and purpose in our lives. It has been found to be a fundamental way of increasing our own positivity, happiness and wellbeing at the same time, known as the 'helper's high'. A win, right?

As I outlined at the start of Chapter 11, on relationships, we are a social species; helping each other is part of what binds us together. It can increase our sense of belonging and reduce feelings of loneliness. Sadly, though, it feels like our society is currently losing altruism to some degree. We need to bring it back!

What could you do?

I try to consciously do at least one thing a day to help others. It might be picking up another child from school, bringing one of the soccer mums a box of the tea I have been going on about every week, texting a friend who I know is struggling, letting someone with just a few items go in front of me at the supermarket . . . Some days I might end up doing more things; like everything in life, it ebbs and flows, but my *intention* is there and altruism is a habit for me because of that.

ACTION TIME! Could you look for opportunities for random acts of kindness? Volunteer in your community? Take a meal to a friend who is struggling? Give blood? Donate to charity? Check in on your neighbour? Send your friend a random bunch of flowers for no other reason than you think she is awesome?

Every little act of kindness towards another person, however small, adds up. And small things can become big things when they get shared.

'Create a life that feels good on the inside and not just on the outside.'

— Unknown source

Final thoughts

Thank you for being here and sharing your time with me. I know there are millions of books out there to choose from and I feel extremely grateful that you are reading this one. I really hope that this book is the beginning of you being able to see that things can be different, that there is a new story you can create for yourself, and that if you believe in yourself then anything is possible.

Opening up my life and sharing my story has been an emotional ride, especially telling my parents (at age 42) about the self-harm and near-life-ending events I have been through, but it has taught me so much. Mostly that **it is never too late to have hard**

conversations, and it is never too late to face your challenges and work on healing yourself.

I've had to dig deep to write this book, and many times I was tempted to give up because it felt too hard. But I didn't give up, for the simple reason that I finally believe in myself and believe I can make a difference. I have grappled with my demons and come out the other side, lighter and brighter.

My hope for you is that you can do the same.

And I *know* you can. You, too, just have to start to believe in yourself.

Now go chase your dreams and take care of yourself.

I believe in you.

With love,
Claire x

Acknowledgements

To my mum and dad, thank you for your unwavering support and encouragement no matter what.

Mum, I know it has been hard for you to read this book and learn about some aspects of my journey for the first time. Please know that your journey with dieting and body dissatisfaction has now turned full circle into me helping thousands of people improve their relationship with food and themselves, so that they no longer have to struggle like you and I did for so long.

Dad, thank you for teaching me that kindness is what the world needs more than anything, and that supporting others to heal and grow is one of the best gifts you can give. You have always helped me to believe that anything is possible.

To my husband, thank you for your support through the crazy year it was writing this book while renovating our house, working through a relocation and many other ups and downs.

To my boys Zac and Josh, I love you so much. I'm sorry that I missed so many weekends with you while I was working on this book, but your encouragement with 'How many thousands of words left?' each week was in its own (slightly painful) way motivating me to create the space to get it done.

To my incredible team who support me and some of my crazy work ideas — you are the best of the best! Milly, Hayley, Amy and Kate, I can't thank you enough for holding my virtual hand through this process. And to my crew at Mission Nutrition, I am so grateful to have the honour of working with you! Thank you for all that you do.

To my business manager Dean, you are just amazing. You have helped me in more ways than you will ever know, most of all to truly believe in myself and what I am capable of. Thank you for accepting me just as I am.

To my amazing, mind-blowing friends who have patiently waited for me to come out of book-writing hibernation and who encouraged me from the sidelines, near and far. I feel your love always and it keeps me going more than you'll ever know.

Finally, to you. Thank you for taking a chance and buying this book to explore my thoughts and ideas. I hope this is the beginning of a wonderful journey for you.

Additional reading and resources

Sleep
- www.sleepfoundation.org
- Find out what chronotype you are: go to https://qxmd.com/calculate and search on 'morningness'
- Book: *Why we sleep: The new science of sleep and dreams*, Matthew Walker (Allen Lane, 2017)

Nutrition
- Mission Nutrition: www.missionnutrition.co.nz
- My own website for tools and support: www.claireturnbull.co.nz
- Division of responsibility approach with children: www.ellynsatterinstitute.org
- Alcohol: www.alcohol.org.nz

Movement

- Kate Ivey: www.kateiveyfitness.com

Stress management

Mindfulness apps:

- Calm: www.calm.com
- Headspace: www.headspace.com
- Insight Timer: www.insighttimer.com

Relationships

- John Gottman: www.gottman.com
- Esther Perel: www.estherperel.com

Perimenopause/menopause

- Australasian Menopause Society: www.menopause.org.au
- Niki Bezzant: www.nikibezzant.com (check out her 'Article library' and books)
- Dr Jen Gunter: @drjengunter, https://drjengunter.com/
- Dr Mary Claire Haver: @drmaryclaire

Trauma

- Book: *The body keeps the score: Brain, mind, and body in the healing of trauma*, Bessel van der Kolk (Viking, 2014); also www.besselvanderkolk.com
- Book: *The myth of normal: Trauma, illness, and healing in a toxic culture*, Gabor Maté with Daniel Maté (Avery, 2022); also www.drgabormate.com

Addiction

- Book: *Dopamine Nation: Finding balance in the age of indulgence*, Anna Lembke (Dutton, 2021); also www.annalembke.com

- Book: *The molecule of more: How a single chemical in your brain drives love, sex, and creativity — and will determine the fate of the human race*, Daniel Z. Lieberman and Michael E. Long (BenBella Books, 2018)

Mental health helplines

- Need to talk? Free call or text 1737 any time for support from a trained counsellor
- Lifeline — 0800 543 354 (0800 LIFELINE) or free text 4357 (HELP)
- Youthline — 0800 376 633, free text 234 or email talk@youthline.co.nz or online chat
- Samaritans — 0800 726 666
- Suicide Crisis Helpline — 0508 828 865 (0508 TAUTOKO)
- Depression Helpline — 0800 111 757 or free text 4202 (to talk to a trained counsellor about how you are feeling or to ask any questions)
- EDANZ — improving outcomes for people with eating disorders and their families. Freephone 0800 2 EDANZ or 0800 233 269, or in Auckland 09 522 2679. Or email info@ed.org.nz
- Healthline — 0800 611 116. Health advice from professional healthcare providers
- Alcohol and Drug Helpline — 0800 787 797 or online chat
- Are You OK (family violence helpline) — 0800 456 450
- Gambling Helpline — 0800 654 655 or free text 8006
- Anxiety NZ — 0800 269 4389 (0800 ANXIETY)

Psychologists

Tools for finding a psychologist:

- www.nzccp.co.nz/for-the-public#find-a-psychologist
- www.psychology.org.nz/public/find-psychologist

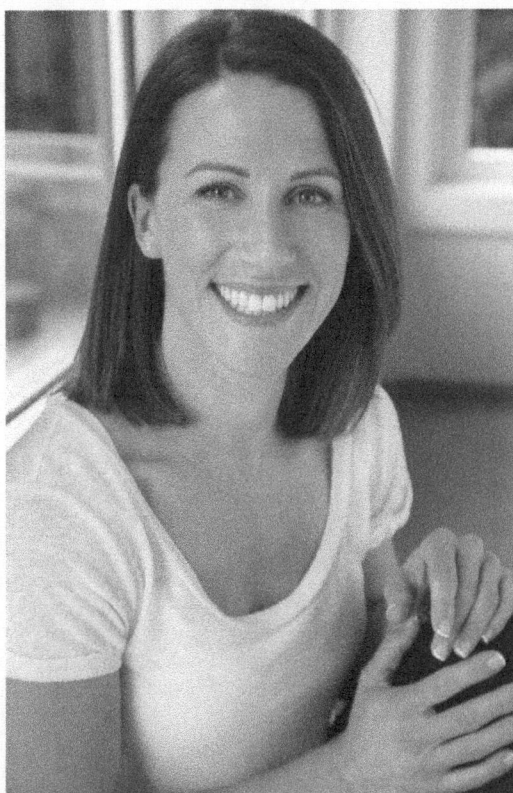

About the author

Claire Turnbull is a registered nutritionist with a diploma in positive psychology. She is the founder of Mission Nutrition and the author of two previous books on wellbeing.

Originally from the United Kingdom, Claire has called New Zealand home for more than two decades. She lives with her husband and two children in Queenstown.